GETTING READY GUIDE

DUE DATE

EVERYTHING YOU NEED TO KNOW ABOUT YOUR PREGNANCY JOURNEY

DR. SUNIL KUMAR G S
MD, DNB, FRCR (UK)

STARDOM BOOKS

STARDOM BOOKS

WORLDWIDE

www.StardomBooks.com

STARDOM BOOKS

A Division of Stardom Publishing

and infoYOGIS Technologies.

105-501 Silverside Road

Wilmington, DE 19809

Copyright © 2021 by Dr. Sunil Kumar G S

All rights reserved, including right to reproduce
this book or portions thereof in any form whatsoever

FIRST EDITION OCTOBER 2021

Stardom Books

Getting Ready Guide
DUE DATE
Everything You Need to Know About
Your Pregnancy Journey

Dr. Sunil Kumar G S

p. 270
cm. 13.5 X 21.5

Category: Health & Fitness / Pregnancy &
Childbirth

ISBN-13: 978-1-7369486-8-2

DEDICATION

To all my readers, teachers, and well-wishers
To my wife Sharadhi, who is a mother of two daughters, and has been an inspiration to write this book
To the entire medical fraternity
To members of add-on Scans and Labs.

CONTENTS

A Bag Full of Gratitude	i
FOREWORD	iii
PRAISE FOR THE BOOK	v
INTRODUCTION	1

PART 1: THE BEGINNING OF THE JOURNEY

1	ARE YOU READY FOR THE PREGNANCY?	7
2	PREPARING TO BECOME PREGNANT	13
3	AM I PREGNANT? SHOULD I CONTINUE THE PREGNANCY?	19
4	CHOOSING THE RIGHT DOCTOR	25
5	HOW TO COPE WITH THE DISCOMFORTS OF PREGNANCY?	29
6	ROLE OF THE FATHER-TO-BE	35

PART 2: ESSENTIALS OF PREGNANCY

7	EATING RIGHT IN PREGNANCY	43
8	FITNESS DURING PREGNANCY	55
9	PRENATAL YOGA	59
10	REST AND SLEEPING POSTURE	69

11	WORK AND TRAVEL DURING PREGNANCY	73
12	SKIN CARE DURING PREGNANCY	79
13	MENTAL HEALTH DURING PREGNANCY	83

PART 3: PRENATAL TESTING

14	ULTRASOUND SCAN DURING PREGNANCY	89
15	PRENATAL GENETIC TESTS IN PREGNANCY	95
16	AMNIOCENTESIS AND CHORIONIC VILLUS SAMPLING	101

PART 4: YOUR PREGNANCY CALENDAR: MONTH ON MONTH

FIRST TRIMESTER

17	PREGNANCY CALENDAR: FIRST MONTH	107
18	PREGNANCY CALENDAR: SECOND MONTH	109
19	PREGNANCY CALENDAR: THIRD MONTH	119

SECOND TRIMESTER

20	PREGNANCY CALENDAR: FOURTH MONTH	123
21	PREGNANCY CALENDAR: FIFTH MONTH	127
22	PREGNANCY CALENDAR: SIXTH MONTH	133

THIRD TRIMESTER

23	PREGNANCY CALENDAR: SEVENTH MONTH	139
24	PREGNANCY CALENDAR: EIGHTH MONTH	145

25	PREGNANCY CALENDAR: NINTH MONTH	153
26	MILESTONES ACCOMPLISHED AT EVERY MONTH	159
27	LABOR AND DELIVERY	163
28	CESAREAN SECTION	169
29	CORD-BLOOD SAMPLING	175

PART 5: AFTER DELIVERY

30	NEWBORN CARE	179
31	BIRTH CONTROL AFTER DELIVERY	189
32	BREASTFEEDING	195

PART 6: COMMON ISSUES IN PREGNANCY

33	MULTIPLE PREGNANCY	199
34	GESTATIONAL DIABETES	203
35	HYPERTENSION IN PREGNANCY	207
36	FETUS GROWTH RESTRICTION	211
37	UNDERSTANDING MISCARRIAGE AND COPING WITH IT	213
38	PRETERM LABOR AND DELIVERY	219
39	CERVICAL INCOMPETENCE	223
40	ECTOPIC PREGNANCY	225
41	RH INCOMPATIBILITY	227

42	COMMON ISSUES IN PREGNANCY	229
43	COMMON INFECTIONS IN PREGNANCY	233
44	FIBROIDS	237
45	GETTING PREGNANT AFTER 35 YEARS	239
	CONCLUSION	241

A BAG FULL OF GRATITUDE

Writing a book on pregnancy is easy either for a Gynecologist or a pregnant woman. As I am a Fetal Radiologist, I do not fall into either of these categories. However, I decided to write a book on pregnancy when I realized that I am supported by many people who are experts either in the subject of childbirth or other related fields. Hence, I am opening up my bag of gratitude to all those who had given me a hand when I needed them on my writing journey.

Let me pick up the 'gratitudinal' gifts that I have kept aside for Dr. Sangeetha D. Gomes, Dr. Archana Pathak, Dr. Puja Rathi, Dr. Aruna Kumari, Dr. Nupur Sood, Dr. Jyoti Kala, Dr. Harsha V. Reddy, Dr. Triveni M.P., Dr. Anupama Rani, Dr. Dhivya Chandrasekar, and Dr. Mohammed Rishard, who are my Gynaecology friends. They have freely shared their valuable inputs and experiences, which form the crux of this book. The next set of gifts are set aside for Dr. Lini Balakrishnan, Pediatrician; Dr. Sapna R. Revankar, Dermatologist; and Dr. Sharanabasavaraj, Psychiatrist; who have contributed their thoughts in the chapters on "Newborn Care", "Skin Care," and "Mental Health," respectively.

Despite his busy schedule, Mr. Ryan Fernando, the celebrity Nutritionist, has contributed an entire chapter on "Eating Right in Pregnancy" for the well-being and health of expectant mothers. Hence, I offer great thanks to him for the valuable service he has given me. Physio Meghana Dave and Mrs. Priya Nair have given ample inputs on fitness and prenatal yoga. I thank them for their work.

I am indebted to Mr. Sunil Jain from Astha Foundation for holding me accountable and pushing me to complete the project on time. My wholehearted gratitude to Mr. Suresh Babu for his support and guidance. I cannot restrain myself from thanking Mr. Raam Anand, a good friend and the publisher of this book, for his unconditional support. Mrs. Achu Anna Mathew has been instrumental in the creation of this book. I extend my gratitude to these wonderful people for backing me up whenever I needed help.

I am deeply indebted to my wife Sharadhi Suresh and my family members for being strong foundations of moral and emotional support. I thank my colleagues Dr. Mamatha R., Dr. Shilpa Chaitanya Reddy, and Dr. Elluru Santhosh for encouraging me to write this book. I extend my thanks to all the members of 'add-on Scans &Labs' for their unconditional support and for providing me with ample time by taking up some of my responsibilities, which has been a great help in bringing out this book.

FOREWORD

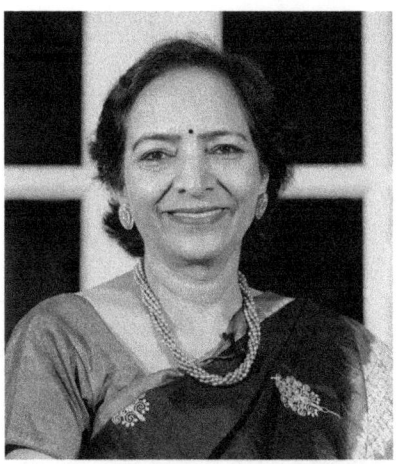

This book called "Due Date" is very aptly named because of the uncertainty of the time at which the baby decides to come out. I would like to say that the very fact this book has interviews of many pregnant women with various symptoms, here the author has taken the trouble to analyze this and put it into a scientific manner and hence it requires to be applauded. Most of the time doctors tend to give a purely scientific explanation which may not go down well with pregnant women. A large number of stories in this book pick up the symptomatic issues of pregnant women and gives a scientific basis for them. This book should be a must-read for women as it is sure to give them the necessary peace and comfort at a time when they need, perhaps in the middle of the night, when their anxiety is high and the doctor is unavailable. I look forward to seeing this book as a ready reckoner on the mantelpiece of every pregnant mother and wish this due date when it comes, is a very happy occasion for both the mother and the obstetrician. I congratulate Dr Sunil Kumar for this enterprise and I hope many more such books will come from him. I wish him all the success.

Thank you very much

Padma Shri Dr Kamini A Rao

PRAISE OF THE BOOK

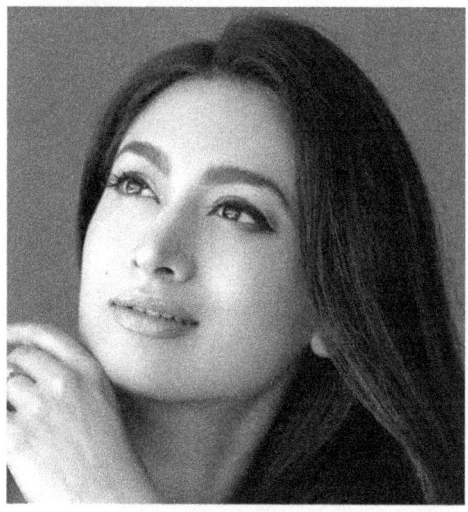

This brilliant book is a boon for expectant mothers. When I read about the book, all I could think was: *"This book would have been of such a great help when I was carrying, or even before I decided to get pregnant."* I could relate to so many instances from this book; all of them are so relevant.

I must say, this book details every aspect of your pregnancy, right from preparing for pregnancy till motherhood, and that is the beauty of this book.

I strongly recommend this book and perhaps would not think twice to gift this book to an expectant mother or anybody planning to conceive. I want to thank Dr. Sunil for his contribution from the bottom of my heart. I'm sure this book will help millions out there as it busts all myths and misconceptions around pregnancy and delivery. Kudos to Dr. Sunil Kumar!

Shwetha Srivatsav
(Actress and mom-vlogger)

INTRODUCTION

Are you pregnant? Or are you planning to get pregnant? If so, this book will be your buddy throughout your pregnancy journey. When my wife conceived our second daughter, I decided to gift her some pregnancy books that she could use during her journey. She was overwhelmed by the medical jargon and the size of the books and helplessly asked me how she could read them all. She wondered if I could write a book on pregnancy that laymen could easily understand.

This made me pause for thought, and I could definitely write a book on pregnancy, even though I only have second-hand experience in dealing with pregnancies. I would often find my wife looking for information on the Internet rather than referring to the book I had given her whenever she had a doubt.

However, she often complained that it was easy to get lost in the vast information that was available on the Internet. As she was nearing her due date for delivery, she once commented that she could now advise her friends, the would-be mothers, on the different changes that they can expect in their bodies during pregnancy and offer tips for them to follow.

Even though she is a non-medical person, she informed me that she seriously plans to start a pregnancy counseling clinic for expectant mothers after delivery. This made me curious, and I asked her what gave her this different idea. She replied that pregnant women would never take time to read those enormous books, and if she could provide insights from her own pregnancy, that would be a first-hand experience from a once pregnant lady.

She also mentioned that they could avoid checking the Internet and enjoy this peaceful phase in their life, rather than getting lost in the vast amount of data found online. This struck an idea, and I asked her what her opinion was about writing a guide for pregnant women. She was excited about the idea, but also a little anxious that it should not be yet another difficult-to-read voluminous book on pregnancy like those already in the market. I asked her for suggestions on how the book ought to be.

She suggested that it should be an interesting book, more like a storybook or novel, which women could easily read. She gave me the idea of including various case stories that I have discussed with her about the different pregnant women that I have encountered. Those stories were really interesting and helpful to her, as she could relate their condition to hers. So, here I am with a pregnancy book, *Due Date*, which will help you refer to the different concepts associated with pregnancy quickly.

The term *Due Date* might bring to your mind concepts such as labor, delivery, Cesarean section, etc. However, here, I am trying to portray the journey from conception till birth and afterward. One of the recurring and the most often asked questions that I encounter during the pregnancy scans is, "When is my due date?". Pregnant women are always excited about this phase in their lives and repeatedly ask me the same question whenever they come for their routine scans. Hence, when I started writing the book, the first word that came to my mind for the title was *Due Date*, although it is a misnomer, because only four percent of pregnant women deliver on the due date.

I have shared many case stories in this book so that my readers can relate their own conditions to the stories they read. Moreover, stories are easier to remember than a regular lecture or a description of the condition. However, information on all the conditions I mention in the book is available on the Internet. I have just tried to pen down some issues which are commonly expressed by pregnant women.

In fact, I prefer to call my book a reference guide for couples who are devoid of parental support. As every experience they face during their pregnancy journey is new to them, I hope this book will give them a clear insight into their pregnancy. However, I wish to remind my readers that the experience of pregnancy is different for different individuals.

That is why I have attempted to explain the situations with multiple case-based stories that could be applicable to normal and abnormal pregnancy conditions. In this book, many Obstetricians and Gynecologists have provided valuable inputs from their expertise and experiences in dealing with pregnancy. Hence, this book is a culmination of ideas and inputs from various Doctors and related healthcare professionals. Along with multiple inputs from multiple people, I have tried to incorporate the latest practice in medicine associated with pregnancy.

Please take note that these inputs and suggestions are personal views, and hence, you have the choice of accepting them or not. My book is a guide and not a treatment manual. Kindly consider this as a guide only, as it is not my intention to recommend any treatment procedure.

Hence, if you experience an abnormal change in your body during pregnancy, I advise you to consult your Doctor for further treatment procedures. The ideas that I have portrayed in the book are very general and may apply to many circumstances you experience, but not all.

This book gives a bird's eye view of the pregnancy journey, and let me tell you something very important. The content on pregnancy is exhaustive, and hence it was difficult for me to compile all the concepts in a single book. In fact, I did not want it to be a voluminous book that is packed with so many facts and medical literature.

I know that my readers will lose interest if I produce a book like that. If you feel that I have not analyzed the different pregnancy conditions in-depth, please understand that this book is not medical literature. I intended to provide glimpses on pregnancy and make my readers read the book very easily.

Most of the pregnancies are uneventful; hence, this book covers mostly the physiological changes and the common discomforts and issues faced by the pregnant woman, and can be a guide on what to expect when you are pregnant. I am sure that the pregnant women who read my pregnancy guide would be able to relate the case stories that I have presented in my book with their current conditions. I know that pregnancy comes with many doubts and questions and many pregnant women are eager to ask these questions to their respective Doctors. Even I have encountered questions from many pregnant women when they approach me for their routine scans.

In our current scenario, Doctors have a fully packed schedule, with an enormous amount of duty, and hence, most often, time does not permit them to answer all the queries of the patients. I hope this book will act as a problem-solver or a counselor when traveling through the most significant phase of your life.

Pregnant women are not termed patients as pregnancy is considered a physiological process, and not as something abnormal. However, in some chapters, I have used the term patients. Kindly bear with me for describing them thus in some parts.

The patient names mentioned in the case stories are not factual, and hence, any resemblance you feel is just a coincidence.

As the last pointer, I would like to mention that diet, fitness, and travel form the major part of pregnancy. I have given enough emphasis to these areas in order to portray their importance.

I hope these pointers will help you in having an insightful and joyous pregnancy journey. I wish my readers all the best for their pregnancy, and I hope that my book will help navigate you toward your due date.

PART 1

PART 1

1

ARE YOU READY FOR PREGNANCY?

Motherhood is one of the most precious roles a woman could embrace in her life. I recently read a quote on motherhood by the famous Lebanese author Sandra Chami Kassis: "You never understand life until it grows inside of you". If you are reading this book, you must be going through this phase in your life or preparing to become a mother.

I have seen many couples struggle to get pregnant even after undergoing several treatments. One of the major misconceptions among married couples is that pregnancy will occur naturally. According to a study conducted on married women by *FPA, a sexual health company, around 30 percent got pregnant just a month after marriage.

Furthermore, 75 percent became pregnant within the first six months, and almost 90 percent of them were pregnant within one year. These cases fall under the natural conception method, where sexual relations between the husband and the wife led to pregnancy, which was not aided by any medication. However, the remaining 10 percent of these women needed more time. The association did a study on these women to understand this delay in their conception.

One major issue they found was the unreadiness of accepting a new family member's arrival. Unless your mind and body are ready to accept the pregnancy, you will not be able to conceive even if you have undertaken many treatment procedures. I had a patient struggling to get pregnant, and after taking treatment for five years, she finally became pregnant.

Upon inquiry, she revealed her heart-breaking story. She and her husband were married for 11 years. At first, there were no issues between them, as they thought that pregnancy would happen naturally. Both of them were working professionals in multinational companies (MNCs) and had tight schedules. After six years of marriage, they realized that there could be some underlying issues as she was unable to conceive. So, they consulted a Doctor, and both of them underwent thorough check-ups.

However, the Doctor could not find any problem with either the husband or the wife. So, the Doctor prescribed ovulation-inducing medicines to the woman for three consecutive cycles. However, even after following the medication plan, she was not able to conceive. As a last resort, they opted for in vitro fertilization (IVF) treatment. They approached an infertility center and underwent the IVF procedure thrice. However, even this proved to be futile, and the couple was left devastated. People around them, including family members and friends, branded the wife as infertile and barren. After two years, they again met a Gynecologist, who advised them to take a break from work and try again with medication. They finally succeeded in getting pregnant. Both of them were ready to accept the baby physically and mentally. Previously, the severe work pressure had wreaked havoc on their mental state, and they had not been emotionally ready to accept the pregnancy.

So, at this point, let us take a closer look into the different aspects of readiness. Being ready for pregnancy means your mind and body should be prepared to accommodate the new life that will grow within you. First, let us look at the aspects of the mind. Pregnancy is a condition that creates many hormonal imbalances, which can sometimes topple the mental state of a mother-to-be. It is a stage when you find yourself being upset even over trivial matters. For example, you may find yourself crying while watching a television episode where the mother-in-law mistreats her daughter-in-law. You may be perplexed by your tears and wonder why you shed tears. However, do not blame your emotions alone.

It is the increase of estrogen and progesterone that causes these mood swings. This tendency is evident in the first trimester as these hormones will rapidly increase to prepare the body for pregnancy. Irritability is also an accompanying emotion that you find in pregnant women. It is usual to find a pregnant woman indulging in issues emotionally. Hence, do not beat yourself. Instead, try to understand the condition, which has a lot to do with the mood swings.

Sometimes, these irritable and sad emotions might end up being dangerous. Once I was asked to attend to a patient who was six months into her pregnancy. She accidentally fell while watching a movie. Her husband and parents were afraid for her and her baby's condition as she fell on her tummy. When I asked her about the incident, she said that she was watching the Bahubali movie while eating apples. When she saw Devasena being captured by Ballaladeva, she stood up anxiously. She told me how she accidentally stood up on the wet floor that was mopped a second before the incident and slipped. Somehow, she was lucky that nothing happened to the baby. I assured her and her family that the baby was fine and healthy inside the womb.

Emotional imbalances often create certain accidents, which sometimes turn out to be dangerous. Women often experience mood swings during the premenstrual syndrome (PMS); however, the mood swings experienced during pregnancy might be more severe. A growing baby inside the womb calls for many adjustments and restrictions on the mother's part.

You cannot enjoy your favorite delicacies, as you will be more vulnerable to diet-related issues like raised blood pressure and Diabetes. Likewise, you might not be able to travel as you used to. So, getting ready for pregnancy means you have to be mentally prepared for the adjustments you need to make during the 40 weeks of pregnancy. Just like mental readiness, your body should also be ready to accept the baby.

The first element in physical readiness comes with maintaining a healthy weight. Your body weight is always connected to your lifestyle. The healthier the lifestyle is, the healthier the weight will be. Being overweight is often linked with Poly-Cystic Ovarian Disorder (PCOD) and thyroid issues. It is like a triangular phenomenon where PCOD, hypothyroidism, and obesity occupy the three corners. Being overweight has been a major stumbling block in the lives of many women.

So, before you prepare to become pregnant, make sure to have an ideal weight and an ideal lifestyle. Weight management is done with the help of exercise and diet. It is good to take advice from an expert Nutritionist on diets for weight reduction. The Nutritionist will make sure that you are consuming enough nutrients to keep your body healthy. Before conceiving, the Doctors might also prescribe medicines like folic acids, vitamins, calcium, iron tablets, etc.

Pregnancy is a time when you will have many cravings. Sometimes you may wish to eat junk food, which most Doctors would want you to avoid. Junk food is not nutritious, and consuming it might increase your chance of gaining more weight. Other hormonal issues will also accompany the enormous consumption of junk foods.

Home-made food, which is very nutritious, should be part of your diet. You can garnish healthy food according to your cravings and tastes. However, if you have Diabetes or have been detected to have Gestational Diabetes in your previous pregnancies, you should restrict the sugar intake to avoid complications during pregnancy.

One of the crucial things you ought to do if you are preparing for pregnancy is to detoxify your body. It is best to stop consuming alcohol and limit your caffeine intake as these affect the quality of the egg and sperm; alcohol and caffeine can also affect your regular sleep cycle. Ensure that you get sufficient sleep if you are preparing for pregnancy. Lack of sleep leads to tiredness, which is a significant obstacle to conception. This lack of rest might sometimes alter the woman's ovulation pattern, which adds to the difficulty in conceiving.

I had a patient named Veena, who was an Assistant Vice President in an MNC. Her Gynecologist suspected that she might have PCOD and wanted to get an ultrasound scan. I could not find any issues in her scan images. Out of curiosity, I asked her about her diet and rest patterns.

As she was a top executive in the company, she hardly got time to take any rest. She was also in the habit of drinking more than 10 cups of coffee daily to remain awake.

Additionally, due to her regularly attending company parties and gatherings, she consumed alcohol often. I hinted that this lifestyle might be the reason for her incapability to get pregnant. After two years, she came back for her early pregnancy scan. She was able to conceive once she changed her lifestyle.

I asked her about her work and busy schedules, and she replied that she had taken a short break to get completely ready for the pregnancy. That was an eye-opener for me. Even though she had reached such a high level in the company hierarchy, she took a break to prepare for pregnancy fully. Exercise is another vital practice associated with pregnancy. Exercise helps you maintain the optimum weight and aids you in getting pregnant.

Some studies on pregnant women have revealed that moderate exercises like jogging, walking, biking, etc., are associated with a shorter conception period. Adopt a regular exercise regime for easier and faster conception. The habit of smoking can also lead to negative results. It does not matter whether you are an active smoker or a passive smoker. It is always advisable to quit smoking when you are planning a pregnancy. It would be best to adopt all these practices when you start thinking about extending your family. I have given you an outlook on how to be physically and mentally ready for your pregnancy.

Now, I would like to share a few thoughts on emotional readiness. Usually, we think emotional readiness and mental readiness are the same. However, it is vital to know that both concepts are different and that there is only a thin line between them. Parenthood is a responsibility that should not be weighed by emotions alone.

I have seen many parents, especially those who had to wait a long time for a baby, overlook their children's wrongdoings. I believe that this is not exclusively true as it ultimately depends on the baby's upbringing. Every parent should have proper emotional readiness, enabling them to accept their baby as an ordinary being, just like anyone else's. Another primary concept associated with emotional readiness lies in the couple's capacity to accept all the physical and mental changes that might happen before, during, and after pregnancy.

The couple should also be aware of postpartum depression that might hinder the relationship between them. All these facts should be considered when you start thinking about pregnancy. Many couples consider rearing a baby to be a burden, wherein they always forget that a baby is the true binding force between the husband and the wife. Apart from that, babies are the light that dawns upon the family throughout their life. Now, the question that remains is, are you really ready for pregnancy?

If the answer is yes, what are the preparations you have done to welcome the new member of the family? In the next chapter, let us discuss the different preparations you have to make mentally, emotionally, and physically, which will enable you to have a calm and composed pregnancy experience.

2

PREPARING TO BECOME PREGNANT

Pregnancy is divided into three trimesters, with each trimester having a duration of at least 13 weeks. That means each trimester spans three months. Out of these, the first month is the phase of the advent of the good news.

In the first month, some people are unaware of the changes happening in their bodies, whereas some can easily identify the signs and symptoms of pregnancy.

One of my old colleagues, Dr. Radhika, told an interesting story during our family get-together. She is a Gynecologist working in a reputed hospital in Bengaluru. One of her patients complained about a positive pregnancy test when she did not exhibit any pregnancy signs. She had mild bleeding, which led her to believe that her hemoglobin might be low, and hence she experienced menstruation that had a "shortage of blood."

Dr. Radhika too suspected pregnancy as the pregnancy test was positive. However, it was tough to convince the patient. Finally, she asked the patient to go for a Beta–human chorionic gonadotrophin (Beta-hCG) test and ultrasonography to confirm the pregnancy and end the heated argument.

As expected, she was six weeks pregnant. Dr. Radhika concluded her story by revealing that many women might not experience pregnancy signs and symptoms early in pregnancy. I remember meeting a woman named Reshma, who narrated a similar story to me. She felt tired and thought that it could be due to the challenging nature of her work at her office. As she could not get rid of the tiredness, she thought of visiting a Doctor. She was not expecting to be pregnant as her periods were not regular.

As her husband was a Colonel in the Army, she went to meet the Army Doctor on her bicycle. She was surprised to learn that she was six weeks pregnant and gazed at her bicycle in dismay. Sometimes negligence and ignorance might cause complications.

When you are ready to accept the pregnancy, you should start preparing your body for it. Are you aware of the major things you should know while preparing for pregnancy? First, you should stop using birth control measures: once you stop using birth control measures and start indulging in sexual contact during the ovulation period, the chances of becoming pregnant are high. A good diet is essential always for a healthy outcome of pregnancy. However, it is misinterpreted in many ways.

A good diet is not synonymous with increased food quantity; instead, it means a healthy and balanced diet. For example, it is always better to consume whole food than processed food, and if you include organic food in your diet, it will definitely be more beneficial. If you are planning for a baby, you must remain healthy. Hence, it is essential to get your vitals checked regularly.

Ensure to check these basic blood parameters before conceiving.

- Thyroid hormone levels
- Blood sugar levels
- Cholesterol levels
- Hemoglobin level

If you have issues like thyroid hormone deficiency, high cholesterol levels, or Diabetes, it might affect you and your baby. One of my friends had three consecutive miscarriages. She was the mother of a three-year-old baby and was planning for another. During her third miscarriage, her Gynecologist asked her if she had checked her thyroid hormone levels before conceiving.

She never had any symptoms of thyroid dysfunction, but as her Doctor had advised, she decided to get it checked. The Doctor was surprised to find that she had high levels of thyroid stimulating hormone (TSH).

According to the American Thyroid Association, the reference range for TSH in the different phases of pregnancy are as follows:

- First trimester: 0.1–2.5 µIU/mL
- Second trimester: 0.2–3.0 µIU/mL
- Third trimester: 0.3–3.0 µIU/mL.

She was prescribed medication, and after one year, she had her second baby. After the delivery, she went to meet her Doctor. After coming back from the Doctor, she started giving me a class on thyroid hormone and the role it plays in pregnancy. Make sure to take any vaccinations that may have lapsed.

It is essential to take vaccinations for rubella and tetanus while you are planning for the pregnancy. If pregnant women are afflicted with rubella, the chances of a miscarriage and stillbirth are high.

On the other hand, the tetanus vaccination will safeguard the mother and baby from maternal and neonatal tetanus.

Always schedule a preconception visit to your Gynecologist. You may face hurdles in conceiving depending upon your age, weight, hormonal issues, etc. In such cases, your Doctor will help you overcome these issues. Remember to take your blood and scan reports for such visits. It would help if you consistently track your menstrual cycles to understand your fertile days clearly. I have seen many patients complaining about irregular cycles and issues related to ovulation.

Many women are not aware of the importance of the menstrual cycle and ovulation. Ovulation is the process wherein the ovaries release the egg. If you have a regular 28-day to 30-day cycle, ovulation usually happens between the 12th and 14th days. Most women who complain about irregular cycles will have cycles less than 21 days or more than 35 days. You may say that calculating the ovulation period can be a burden, especially for those with irregular cycles. Refer to the ovulation calculator calendar on the Internet—it is not a difficult science. Let us look at how we could calculate it more easily.

Ovulation always happens 14 days before the next menstrual cycle. Once you master tracking the menstrual cycle, the road to pregnancy becomes clearer. The next step is to start practicing stress-relief methods as stress affects the growth and safety of the baby in the womb. Some stress-relieving habits are practicing yoga and engaging in artistic works.

Pregnancy hormones affect the teeth and the gums. Good dental habits, along with regular visits to the dentist, will help women fight against gingivitis and cavities during pregnancy. Be aware of your family health history. The genetic makeup of the family members will have a strong influence on the baby's health. Hence, if you find some genetic issues or health conditions that trouble you, it is always good to discuss those issues with your Doctor.

I met a patient named Arya, who came for her Nuchal Translucency scan, usually taken during the first trimester, to detect chromosomal abnormalities. We had a wonderful conversation during the entire scanning procedure, in which she asked so many questions related to pregnancy and the baby's growth inside the womb. I then realized that many people were unaware of these facts when they planned for pregnancy.

Maybe you might have learned about these facts when you were in school. A deeper understanding will help you enjoy your pregnancy with much less stress.

Recently, I met a pregnant woman named Radhika, who came for her early pregnancy scan. Everything was normal, and the gestational sac was also visible. So, I showed her the sac during the scanning and mentioned that everything was normal. She was thrilled and asked me if she had twins in her womb. There was only one gestational sac, and it was clear that she had only one baby. I informed Radhika that it was a single baby.

She started crying and asked me if the second baby was dead. I showed her the scan again and explained that she had only one baby within her. I was curious and asked her why she was so confident that she was carrying twins. I was stunned when she told me that she had been consuming ripe twin plantains from the very first day of her marriage to give birth to twins. Many such false beliefs and myths exist about pregnancy, and more so about multiple pregnancies. When you are pregnant, you should start taking multivitamins and folic acid supplements as the nutrients in your body will be sucked up by the growing baby.

Hence, Doctors advise their patients to take these supplements from when they begin thinking about having a baby. I hope you now have greater clarity about preparing for pregnancy. So, once you prepare for pregnancy and become pregnant, the next troubling question is whether to continue with the pregnancy or not. Let us discuss this question in the next chapter.

3

AM I PREGNANT? SHOULD I CONTINUE THE PREGNANCY?

'The wait' is the next phase, where women check for signs and symptoms of pregnancy. It is a phase of excitement for some and a phase of tension for others. I used to ask women about this phase whenever they came for their early pregnancy scans. Many of them said they were quite excited when the home-based pregnancy test showed a positive result. A pregnant woman named Shwetha came for an ultrasound scan as she had missed her periods. She was so worried. Out of curiosity, I asked about the cause of her worry. She had been trying to get pregnant for a while. So, when she missed her periods, the couple were hoping that their efforts had become fruitful. However, the home-based tests showed negative results. So, she decided to get a scan to know more about her condition. The ultrasound scan showed a small fluid space in the uterine cavity, revealing that she was four to five weeks pregnant. However, the baby and its heartbeat were not seen. I told her to present her blood test results, especially serum Beta-hCG, to confirm my findings after correlating with the test results. She was unaware of such tests and later revealed that she had not visited a Gynecologist yet.

She had come for an ultrasound scan on the recommendation of a Physician. I asked her about the home-based tests she took to confirm the pregnancy. She told me that as she was unsure, she used a sugar solution and a salt solution, which was a piece of new information to me. I wonder why people misunderstand the type of tests to confirm pregnancy.

Shwetha's case is not a rarity. I met another woman named Manju, who argued that she was pregnant when her scan report showed the opposite. She tried 10 different natural pregnancy tests, all of which showed different results. She finally consulted an Ayurvedic Doctor, who advised her to undergo an ultrasound scan. After my interaction with her, I realized that it is tough to convince self-declared pregnant women when they are not pregnant. Manju lectured me on the different natural pregnancy tests. She talked of sugar pregnancy tests, salt pregnancy tests, baking soda pregnancy tests, wheat and barley pregnancy tests, mustard powder pregnancy tests, dandelion leaves pregnancy tests, storing urine pregnancy tests, wine pregnancy tests, and tuna juice pregnancy tests, and how all these tests confirmed her pregnancy. The authenticity of these test methods has always been a topic of debate.

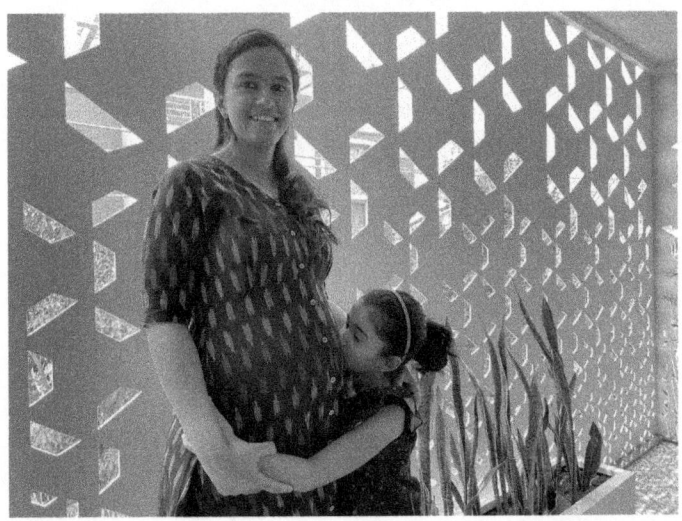

Some of these home pregnancy tests have been in use since ancient times, and are probably still in use to reveal unplanned pregnancies, especially in villages and rural areas.

It is quite natural for women to get anxious when they miss their periods. By that time, some will experience early pregnancy symptoms such as nausea, muscle cramps, fatigue, mood swings, gum bleeding, frequent urination, and excessive thirst and hunger, to name a few. Unfortunately, these symptoms are not unique for everyone. Moreover, many of these symptoms are also associated with PMS and other health conditions.

A patient named Alice came to see me a couple of months back. She was 42 years old and had missed her periods. When she visited a Physician, he suggested that she might have started menopause as pregnancy signs were absent. He instructed her to see a Gynecologist after taking an ultrasound scan for a detailed check-up. She was surprised to know that she was eight weeks pregnant. It was a piece of unexpected news for her as she had not presented any pregnancy signs. This incident should reinforce the truth that one cannot rely on the symptoms alone to confirm pregnancy. **The two reliable ways to confirm pregnancy are the Urine Pregnancy Test (UPT) and the Blood test.** The UPT and the blood test for pregnancy detect the presence of Beta-hCG, a hormone produced during pregnancy, specifically by the developing decidua or placenta. Implantation of the embryo occurs at this phase, and the Beta-hCG hormone gets circulated in the mother's blood.

The Urine Pregnancy Test

It is often referred to as a home pregnancy test or self-testing, the fast, convenient, and cost-effective method to confirm pregnancy. You can collect the UPT kit from any medical store near you without having a prescription. The mother's urine will be analyzed to detect the presence of the hCG hormone. It is always preferable to use the first urine of the day to check for pregnancy.

It should be collected in a dry container for accuracy. You can find two markings C and T (control line and test line) and a space for dropping your urine sample in the kit. You have to put three drops of urine in the area provided and wait for five minutes to get the result. If you find two pink-colored lines near C and T, it means that you are pregnant.

If you see one pink line near the control line, it means you are not pregnant. Furthermore, if there is a pink line in the test line or no pink line in the control line, the test is invalid. It is best if you conduct UPT one week after your missed periods. If the result is negative, and you are still doubtful, you should repeat the test after two days. It is scientifically proven that this test is approximately 99 percent accurate. However, certain conditions like having excessive protein in your body or bloodstains in the urine might provide a false-positive result.

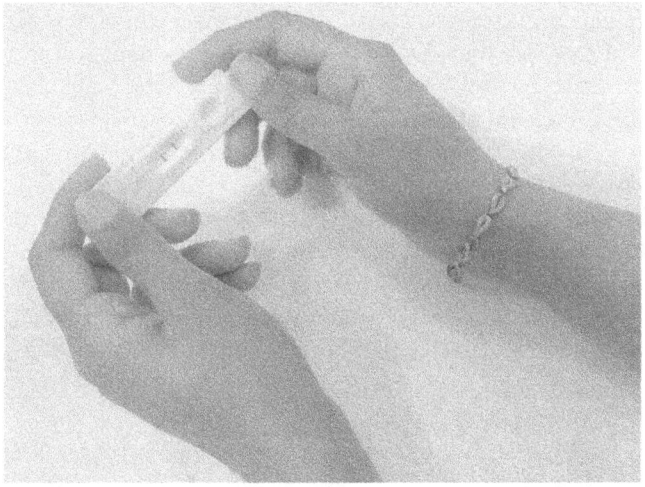

Picture of the UPT kit showing a positive sign for pregnancy.

Serum Beta-hCG

A more reliable method to confirm pregnancy is the blood test, which is said to be 100 percent accurate. This test is called the serum Beta- hCG blood test, where almost 5 mL of your blood is taken for analysis. This test is not the primary test for confirmation. When your Doctor cannot detect the pregnancy by ultrasound scan or suspects an ectopic pregnancy, miscarriage, or molar pregnancy, you will be asked to undertake an hCG test to confirm the pregnancy. Nowadays, many women do the serum Beta-hCG blood tests to be doubly sure of pregnancy. I have seen many cases in which ectopic pregnancies are not identified in the early stages.

A proper consultation with a Physician will help you detect ectopic pregnancies in the beginning stage itself. If left undetected, ectopic pregnancies might cause internal bleeding and infections, and can sometimes be fatal.

Accidental Pregnancy

There are many cases where pregnancy happens without planning. One of the critical questions that may trouble women, in such cases, is whether to continue with the pregnancy. Last year I met a pregnant woman who was carrying her third baby. The couple was not planning for a pregnancy and had been on birth control measures. The woman was 35 years old and was nine weeks pregnant. As they were not interested in another baby, the couple approached a Gynecologist for an abortion.

The Gynecologist objected to their decision and informed them of the side effects. However, the couple was so adamant that they approached another Doctor for the same. I was asked to do a scan the day before the procedure. On hearing the heartbeat of the baby, the mother started crying. Once the scanning was complete, I met her husband and explained his wife's mental strain.

Nevertheless, when I heard that it was the woman who wanted the abortion, I was surprised. I informed the concerned Gynecologist, and she decided to conduct a counseling session for the couple. After the counseling sessions, they decided to move forward with the pregnancy. I was interested in their case and contacted the counselor. She told me that the mother was concerned with how society might view her, especially as she was pregnant for the third time and her eldest daughter was 15 years old. This incident was an epiphany for me.

Many couples have such misapprehensions. However, killing a life is not a solution in such cases. During pregnancy, it is normal to have different feelings. Some women prefer to continue their pregnancy, whereas some decide to terminate it. However, always make sure not to take a hasty decision. Pregnancy hormones might tamper your ability to think rationally. There is another group of women who think of giving up their baby for adoption. The question that should be asked in such situations is "***What changes will happen if I decide to keep my baby?***" Parenting calls for a great deal of responsibility.

This job demands your time and energy, unlike a nine-to-six work schedule in a company. Babies need your care, love, and support in all their day-to-day activities. If you are a first-time parent, you should understand that your life will change drastically with the arrival of a baby. I had an interesting patient named Sumithra, who came for her pregnancy scans regularly.

She came to visit me two years back, with many questions on her mind. Being a Radiologist, I was not able to answer all her queries. She was more concerned about how her life would change with the baby's arrival, and wanted to know if I had a baby. With a smile, I replied that I had a six-year-old daughter. From then onwards, most of her questions centered around the changes that happened in both our lives after our baby's arrival. It was like a rapid-fire round with barely a pause for me to answer.

At last, when I got a space to answer her questions, I had only one answer, "Life is perfect now." She stared at me suspiciously. I smiled back and said, "My life has always been perfect. I have been blessed with caring parents, loving siblings, and a dutiful wife. When our daughter entered our life, we realized we had a greater reason to be happy and love each other. What matters in life is the happiness we have and the happiness we share." She did not have any more questions. The last time I met her, she smiled and commented, "I am really happy now. It seems my happiness will increase within the next seven months". When she indirectly hinted that she was two months pregnant, I could not stop laughing. When you become pregnant, you should concentrate on the happiness part alone.

Once you have decided to continue with the pregnancy, the next step is to find the right Doctor who would care for you and support you during your pregnancy journey. Let us discuss the different points to remember on how to choose the right Doctor for you

4

CHOOSING THE RIGHT DOCTOR

Once your pregnancy is confirmed using the UPT, your next worry will be choosing the right pregnancy care—a good Gynecologist, also known as an Obstetrician, and a good hospital. Some pregnant women consult their Family Physicians at the beginning of the pregnancy. Choosing the right Doctor is crucial; it should be someone who is approachable and good at what they do. Meghana, my sister-in-law, had issues getting pregnant after trying for one year. She consulted Dr. Aruna, who is an acquaintance of mine. After treatment with hormones and ovulation induction, my sister-in-law became pregnant.

Similarly, I met a patient named Anila who was unable to conceive for many years. She and her husband consulted many Doctors who advised them on different types of treatments. None of them was successful, and they finally decided to meet a Doctor in Kerala, as Anila was a native of Kerala. The couple was exhausted by this time. The Doctor from her native place went through their files. She informed them that Anila was perfectly fine, except for a few issues with her menstrual cycle. The Doctor put her on hormone therapy to regularize her cycle and induce ovulation. Within four months, the couple was pregnant.

Anila refers to her Gynecologist as 'the miracle lady.' The medications prescribed by the Doctor had that touch of love and care, and the result was no less than a miracle in Anila's life. The right Doctor should come into your life when you start thinking of pregnancy itself. Do not wait for your pregnancy to choose the right Doctor for your care. A pregnant woman needs several Doctors belonging to different specializations.

Obstetricians (Gynecologists) are the primary Doctors to consult during pregnancy. They are the experts trained to handle pregnancy, labor, and other untoward complications. They are the top-rung Doctors in pregnancy care. It is always good to be under the care of a Gynecologist, especially if you have a high-risk pregnancy—if the pregnant woman is aged above 35 years, has gestational Diabetes, high blood pressure, multiple pregnancies, and/or any pre-existing medical or surgical conditions. You might have chosen a Doctor from Homeopathy, Allopathy, or Ayurveda streams. They all have the basic knowledge of pregnancy care and are certified in prescribing medicines. A few of them are even trained to perform normal vaginal deliveries.

I recall meeting a patient by the name of Sneha, who had come for her anomaly scan. She was suffering from severe dizziness and was planning to meet a Doctor, preferably a Gynecologist. I informed her about the need to consult a Physician. As per my instructions, she visited a Physician and later found that she was struggling with Vertigo. The Physician prescribed her a few medicines, which helped her with her discomforts associated with dizziness. She came back to me and thanked me for my advice. This case is not unique to Sneha alone; it is always good to consult a Family Physician.

In fact, you may consult a Family Physician until your ninth month and then switch to an Obstetrician for the delivery. Another group of medical practitioners associated with pregnancy care are the Midwives. They are trained nurses who are capable of conducting normal deliveries. An experienced nurse is as good as any Doctor in conducting a vaginal delivery. However, you must know that Midwives may not be equipped to handle the complications that may arise or address all your concerns. Choosing the right set of Doctors to help you through your pregnancy has always been a topic of discussion. The below-mentioned tips might come in handy while selecting the best team for the best phase of your life.

1. Ask for recommendations from your family members, friends, colleagues, or even neighbors. It is always good to visit a Doctor with whom you can be comfortable.
2. Look for a few Obstetricians near you and check them out.
3. You can make an informed decision by reading the reviews.
4. If you are stuck and cannot choose the right Doctor, search for a good hospital or a Doctor's clinic nearby. It can be a clinic, hospital, nursing home, or birthing center.
5. Choosing a single-specialty hospital, like a Mother-and-Child Hospital, is recommended if there are no pre-existing health problems. A multi-specialty hospital is good for high-risk pregnancies associated with hypertension, Diabetes, or previous pregnancy complications.
6. When looking at these centers, check the level of intensive care unit (ICU) care these places have for your newborn in case of any untoward complications during delivery. God forbid this situation occurs, but it is always best to be prepared. Check if the center also has a Pediatrician, for there are high chances you might continue to consult a child specialist in the same hospital.
7. You can always choose between consulting a Doctor in a clinic or a primary center. There are certain benefits of consulting a Doctor in a small place, as it is affordable and will save you much money. Remember, the best-known Doctor might not always be good. Although I mentioned earlier about seeking recommendations, you should always make your own decision and choose a Doctor with whom you can be comfortable.

Now, I hope you have understood the importance of choosing the right Doctor. Ensure to make the right decisions for you as well as your baby. One of the major obstacles to a calm and composed pregnancy journey is the discomfort you might experience with the baby's growth inside your womb. In the next chapter, let us discuss the different methods to cope with the discomforts you experience in your pregnancy journey.

5

HOW TO COPE WITH THE DISCOMFORTS OF PREGNANCY?

Pregnancy comes with a lot of bodily discomforts due to elevated hormone levels. All three trimesters feature different discomforts, and the experience varies from woman to woman and pregnancy to pregnancy. I recall meeting a patient named Sujatha who complained about the absence of morning sickness. I was taken aback, and I told her that she was fortunate enough not to be dealing with morning sickness; it is usually considered a discomfort among many women. On inquiry, she informed me that her mother-in-law blamed her for feigning pregnancy as she had no morning sickness. She also told me that since all the ladies in her family had experienced morning sickness, her in-laws were not buying her pregnancy claim.

Among many myths associated with pregnancy, some revolve around the symptoms of pregnancy. "Morning sickness happens only in the morning and disappears after the first three months." "It only happens with your first baby." There are many such myths, but all these claims have been proven wrong. This chapter explains the different discomforts associated with pregnancy and seeks to wipe away the doubts and myths that are associated with it.

Some of the significant and common discomforts experienced in pregnancy include nausea, vomiting, swelling, tiredness, breast tenderness, mood variations, body pain, and food aversions. Let us analyze them one by one. Nausea and vomiting are the two most severe discomforts a pregnant woman might encounter.

Olfaction or the sense of smell will be heightened during pregnancy, and as a result, pregnant women are often triggered by specific odors. Good odors like perfume or a floor cleaner can also become the cause for this set-off. A friend of mine shared how such pleasant odors hindered his travel with his pregnant wife.

Both of them were working together and used to travel together. He said the usual, exciting journey had become a tedious one with the arrival of pregnancy. His wife could not stand the air freshener's odor inside the car, and hence she would always prefer to roll down the windows. On the other hand, an open window is also not safe in cities due to the pollution we witness today. In the end, she finally decided to work from home until she delivered their baby. I am pretty sure many of you might be going through similar situations.

Another reason for nausea and vomiting may be related to gastric issues. The elevated hormones lead to an imbalance in the digestion process, which causes heartburn and chest pain. The solution here is to choose healthy eating practices: eat a lesser quantity but eat more frequently, consume more than 10 glasses of water daily, avoid spicy and oily food, and incorporate fiber-rich and organic food products in your diet.

I remember meeting a three-month pregnant woman who complained of chest pain. The Physician recorded and checked her electrocardiogram (ECG) to rule out any cardiac cause, and she was later sent to me for an ultrasound scan to check if the baby was fine. When asked about her food pattern, she conveyed that she could not comfortably eat or drink due to nausea and vomiting.

I passed this information on to her Gynecologist, who later gave her some tips on healthy eating styles: "Healthy eating should not be a part of pregnancy alone. If you continue this practice, you can fight against all the health hazards that might come your way." A complementary discomfort associated with nausea and vomiting is the aversion toward certain types of food substances.

I met a woman named Sarojam who was thrilled to see the changes in her food patterns during pregnancy. Food that was once distasteful to her ended up being her favorite during her pregnancy.

Pregnancy hormones are indeed the real change makers here. Sarojam was curious about these changes that were happening to her. I explained the process and also informed her about other changes she would be experiencing throughout her pregnancy.

Her curiosity knew no bounds. She was interested in knowing more about pregnancy and asked me about an informative guide to give her a deeper insight into this phase of her life. It was at this moment that I realized the need for such a book in the market. Her question was an eye-opener to me. I was excited to see many people interested in learning about the medical situations associated with pregnancy. This was one of the driving forces that led me to write a book on pregnancy.

Puffiness or swelling experienced in the legs, hands, or face is the next catastrophe you will encounter in your pregnancy. Almost two-thirds of women experience skin puffiness. Here, excessive fluid gets accumulated in their feet, hands, legs, and face. The increased hormones in the body lead to excessive retention of water and salt by the kidneys. If you experience too much swelling, you should immediately inform your Doctor. Sometimes, this can be a sign of pre-eclampsia or pregnancy-induced hypertension. In case of mild swelling of the feet and legs, propping up the legs, soaking the feet in lukewarm water, wearing loose clothes, etc., will reduce the swelling.

However, all the bodily changes, including the discomforts you experience, should be informed to your Doctor at the earliest. I had a patient named Sujatha, who came in regularly for her monthly check-ups. When she came in for her nine-month scanning, I could not recognize her, as she had become puffy. A few parts of her body were unusually swollen. Unaware of conditions like pre-eclampsia or hypertension, Sujatha believed this to be a result of her pregnancy. I advised her family to take Sujatha to a hospital immediately. After three months, she came to see me and thanked me for the advice. She had pre-eclampsia, and when taken to the hospital, they immediately admitted her in the ICU. The Doctors decided to conduct a C-section as soon as possible to save the baby. Hence, it is essential to inform your Gynecologist about all your body's changes when you experience it. Breast tenderness is another discomfort experienced during pregnancy. This is also one of the first signs of pregnancy. However, this can also be a part of PMS. Hence, many women complain of misreading breast tenderness.

Tackling breast tenderness during pregnancy calls for a lot of care and clean habits. Sometimes your breast will feel full and heavier. This happens because the pregnancy hormones are preparing your body for milk secretion. You can reduce this discomfort by changing the type of bra you wear. Consider using a sports bra; it will help minimize the breast's movements and hold it close to the chest. It is also good to apply ice packs on painful areas. Witnessing the baby's growth inside her womb is no cakewalk for a mother.

Pregnant women are often extremely fatigued, and I have seen many of them, even my wife, exhausted once they finish their first trimester. The fatigue you experience reflects the strains you undertake for the well-being of your baby. Going to bed early, delegating work responsibilities, keeping away from unnecessary worries, finding proper solutions to fight anemia, etc., are some practices that will help keep the tiredness away. Anamika, a patient of mine, fainted when she came for her early pregnancy scan. This incident occurred during the initial days of my career as a Doctor; I rushed her to the Emergency Room (ER)when I got the message. Her pulse and oxygen levels were going down, and she had started hyperventilating. The Doctors in the ER gave her oxygen and put her on intravenous fluids.

When she recovered, she told me about the different kinds of pressures she was experiencing, both personally and professionally. She kept getting calls from her office even when she had come for a scan. Her manager was heard shouting at her for not submitting a file. This incident caused Anamika to experience excessive anxiety, which in turn caused a panic attack. Therefore, it will always be best to stay calm and relaxed during pregnancy to avoid unforeseeable events. The subsequent discomfort you may experience in your pregnancy is mood swings. Increasing levels of estrogen and progesterone become the causative agents for an imbalance in the mood. You might often spot pregnant women crying over minor issues. Since mood variations can also occur in PMS, many people do not recognize this as a symptom of pregnancy. In one of the conferences I attended, a Gynecologist spoke about one of her patients dealing with similar mood swings.

The woman had come in with her husband for her third month check-up. The Doctor noticed that the husband appeared to be disturbed about something. On being questioned, the husband complained about his wife's irritating behavior.

Although the Gynecologist tried educating the husband, he was not convinced. He questioned the Gynecologist if those elements that result in mood swings could be removed. Amazed upon his inquiry, the Doctor again explained to him the roles of the various hormones in preparing a woman's body for childbirth. The Gynecologist concluded her story by noting that many husbands consider their wives' mood changes irritating. Well, get this. No man can ever understand the pain and discomfort pregnant women experience in the process of birthing. People around pregnant women must learn to cope with their mood swings. They should understand the changes that a woman goes through during this phase and be considerate toward her.

Pregnant women are advised to eat healthily, get plenty of sleep, spend quality time with their partners, and, most importantly, get the right dose of exercise to maintain a good mood. Body pain is another villain that wreaks havoc on your peaceful phase of pregnancy. Headache is very common. The sudden increase in hormones is the leading cause. Drinking lots of water may help in eliminating this pain. Back pain is also commonly seen; it increases with the baby's growth inside the womb. Adjusting your sitting posture, sleeping on the side, trying heat/cold massages, including physical activity in your daily routine, etc., might help get rid of back pain. I remember meeting a pregnant woman who had come in for her anomaly scan. She complained of severe back pain throughout the procedure and asked what could be the reason.

She was very concerned and kept on asking whether anything abnormal could be seen in the scan. Using medical terminology, I explained to her that the pain was caused by the stretching of ligaments around the womb, and this was known as broad ligament pain. I also checked for other medical issues, such as kidney stones, in the scan. I assured her that mild pain is to be expected as the pregnancy progresses and that she should do stretching exercises and adopt a healthy resting posture. I advised her to consult a Gynecologist and get an opinion on the different medicines she could use to relieve the pain.

Many pregnant women consume pain-relieving medication without consulting their Doctors. This can end up becoming a severe issue as certain medications might hinder the growth of your baby. So, make it a point to consult your Doctor before taking any medicine.

When a pregnant woman is experiencing some discomfort, people around her will usually try to comfort her by saying that the discomforts are quite normal in pregnancy. Remember, these 'people' are not Doctors. Only a Doctor can determine if your discomforts are dangerous or not.

Unchecked issues might pose a danger to both the mother and the baby. Just as in the case of an expectant mother, the would-be father too has many roles to perform before, during, and after pregnancy. Many husbands are unaware of the great responsibilities they have to take up while their wives are pregnant. The next chapter will give you an idea of the roles that ought to be performed by husbands or fathers-to-be when their wives are pregnant.

6

ROLE OF THE FATHER-TO-BE

Have you ever wondered how you could support your partner during pregnancy? Accompanying your wife through the pregnancy journey is an essential task. Even though it is hailed to be a time of excitement, pregnancy and childbirth can also be exhausting physically, socially, and emotionally. Providing a comfort zone by helping your partner in her journey will benefit her and your relationship, and, ultimately, your baby. Pregnant women need much support from their loved ones. The husband's active and supportive behavior can affect the pregnancy outcome. This support also serves to increase the bond between the partners. Women, who are lucky enough to experience their husbands' care, are generally less stressed and much more comfortable with the pregnancy and delivery. Having a supportive partner has been shown to reduce pregnancy complications and has demonstrated positive pregnancy outcomes.

Moreover, research has proved that a husband's active involvement and care during the pregnancy period has a long-lasting and positive impact on the baby's health. Many men are confused about how to be a partner in this journey. Some people uphold the misconception that their role ends with the confirmation of pregnancy.

The truth, however, is that the part of a husband is enhanced after the confirmation. Even though the baby is not yet born, your status of being a father starts. However, during the pregnancy period, this fatherly affection and care are supposed to be bestowed on your partner. For some people, the transformation from a bachelor to a husband and from a husband to a father-to-be might be speedy; this sometimes can be frightening. In such cases, some people get exhausted with the knowledge of pregnancy. There is also another group of people who enjoyed the transformation in a prolonged and steady manner. For them, the positive sign of pregnancy will be an occasion of great joy. Let us look at the supportive care that husbands need to give their pregnant wives during the different stages of pregnancy.

First Trimester:

Supportive care should begin early. Husbands should know how pregnancy could affect the physical and psychological state of women. They should either read about it or learn from their peers. In the first three months, women may experience morning sickness, and husbands need to understand their situation and act accordingly. Just standing by her side and making her feel comfortable is an excellent method of support.

Women may often feel tired and may even experience mood swings. The duty of the husbands in such situations is to calm her down and to entertain her, so that the negative moods can be wiped away. If the husband has a smoking habit, cutting down on smoking will help the pregnant wife. Passive smoking has been shown to cause pregnancy complications.

Husbands should always make it a point to accompany their wives during their monthly visits to the Doctor. They should actively participate in the discussions regarding her condition and always ask questions if they have any doubts. Attending antenatal classes with your wives is crucial as it would educate you and give a positive feeling regarding childbirth.

Husbands should start taking up responsibilities from their wives to provide them with relief and rest. Husbands should also understand that the sexual desires of pregnant women will change with pregnancy, and hence, they should be mentally ready to accept this flexibility.

It is crucial that you engage in discussions with your wife regarding the different roles you both have to play in the future and how you want things to shape up. Such discussions will help the wife understand that you are ready to assume the responsibilities of the new role of a father.

Second Trimester:

The second trimester comes with new signs and symptoms of pregnancy of which you might be unaware. Husbands should make an effort to learn about these pregnancy changes and be aware of clinical appointments and their wives' vitamin supplement intake. He should also be conscious of possible pregnancy complications such as high blood pressure, water bag leak, preterm labor, and bleeding. Women need to undertake physical activities like walking and mild exercise. Husbands should take part in these activities and help them to accomplish their daily exercise goals. Supervise the dietary habits of your wife during pregnancy. Ensure that she consumes organic and healthy food and supplements rather than junk food or food from hotels and fast-food chains.

Third Trimester and Delivery:

The delivery can be physically, mentally, and emotionally challenging for women. Getting ready for the delivery may involve many activities, including selecting clothes for the baby, selecting the place of delivery, and many other things related to the baby's arrival. Husbands should be more sensitive during this phase and should prioritize their wife's choices and support them. You should help your wife maintain a baby movement chart and actively communicate with your unborn baby. This will enable a pregnant woman to prepare herself, as the attachment shown by the father-to-be will boost her confidence. Husbands should also be aware of labor contractions and the signs of labor. Even if your wife is going in for a cesarean section (C-section), you can improve her confidence by mentally and emotionally preparing for that procedure. It is vital to be around her during the latter part of the pregnancy. During labor, you should help her cope with the pain by giving massages, and you may support her to walk around during the early phase of labor.

There are other significant things you could do during the latter stages of labor. Support her decisions regarding pain relief, and help communicate her needs to her care providers. Encourage and support her during the pushing phase by holding her hands and comforting her. A supportive partner's presence can have a positive impact. Moreover, women develop a positive attitude towards their partner and the baby.

After Delivery:

The duty of a husband will not end with the delivery. Post-delivery care provided by the partner is also of utmost importance. Being a husband, you should be protective of your wife and helpful to her after your baby's birth. Create opportunities to congratulate her for enduring the pain and suffering and giving birth to your baby. The post-delivery period is also a highly challenging time for the mother. You should be aware of the post-traumatic effects of delivery and should be able to identify those changes in your wife.

You can also offer your help and support by changing diapers, soothing the crying baby, giving comfort during breastfeeding, etc. Both the parents are supposed to take up the responsibility for a baby's growth, development, and actions. Likewise, the pregnancy journey should be undertaken together where the partners take equal responsibilities and work things out together.

Usually, when a woman becomes pregnant, all the responsibilities that come with the pregnancy are taken up by the woman alone. Likewise, after childbirth, women try to take up all the duties for a growing baby. As the father, it is essential to support your wife through this process of bringing up your baby. It is vital for your wife to know and understand the responsibilities you are taking in this process. I have heard many pregnant women complain about their husbands' lack of responsibility during their pregnancies. It has been scientifically proven that women who have enjoyed a husband's role and responsibility during pregnancy experienced a relaxing and comfortable journey compared to women deprived of this chance. Hence, you must provide comfort, love, and care to your wife during this exhausting journey. A Doctor friend of mine, who is working as a Gynecologist, mentioned that one of the major questions she encounters from first-time mothers-to-be is regarding the best food substances they could consume during pregnancy.

Hence, I thought of including an article on the right kind of food one could consume during pregnancy in this book. In the next chapter, you could listen to the insightful message that the celebrity nutritionist Ryan Fernando has provided on eating the right kind of food during pregnancy.

PART 2

7

EATING RIGHT IN PREGNANCY

One of the major obstacles to eating right during pregnancy is the severe craving for unhealthy food you experience, which can harm your health and that of your baby's.

Let us understand the importance of eating right from a professional nutritionist. He is none other than the celebrity nutrition coach, Ryan Fernando. He advises clients on how to eat scientifically for a better body. His celebrity clients over the years include athletes and film stars.

Over time, the spouses of his clients used to sign up with him as well for a family program on fertility and pregnancy nutrition. As an integrative health coach from the Institute of Integrative Nutrition in New York, USA, Ryan Fernando was taught to acknowledge the client's 'BIOINDIVIDUALITY'. He had once mentioned his life story: "Nine years ago, my wife and I set upon a journey to start a family. She was extremely fit but had PCOD and thyroid hormone fluctuations.

My mother-in-law, a Gynecologist, gave us a lot of nutrition advice. We then went to my wife's Doctor, who also provided advice on what to eat and avoid. This is where I began my serious journey of unraveling the food that a mother needs to eat during pregnancy.

All the pieces of advice provided by the Doctors were general and not specific to my wife's culture, genetic conditions, and lifestyle.

She was recommended to consume a lot of 'paneer'. However, she was allergic to paneer. After a few visits to many Doctors, we only got more confused about what to eat.

I then began to unfurl the protocol for a PREGNANCY DIET for my wife. In reality, nine years ago, QUA NUTRITION clinics under my guidance produced the best nutrition protocol for

a. **Fertility Nutrition and Perfect Weight to Conceive**
Start 1-2 years before planning pregnancy,

b. **Pregnancy Nutrition –**
Each trimester has different nutritional needs for both mother and the baby, and

c. **Post Pregnancy –**
Eating for Weight Loss and Breastfeeding starts immediately after delivery and continues up to 2 years. This is the way you should approach the diet in pregnancy.

Importance of Eating Right in Pregnancy

According to Ryan, eating healthy before and during pregnancy is the highest responsibility of a mother, which is non-negotiable. Most women make changes to their dietary habits once they are pregnant. Nutrition in pregnancy is very significant for the growth and development of the baby and has long-lasting effects on the baby's health.

Research is revealing that most of the diseases we have today may be programmed in the womb. So, not only are you responsible for your baby's future, but even the following two generations can hold you accountable.

Therefore, what you eat now will determine your family tree! Mother's nutrition during pregnancy also helps in fetal programming.

The baby learns the nutritional habits of the mother, which is going to influence the eating pattern of the baby for the rest of its life. Therefore, nutrition during pregnancy is vital and significantly impacts the new life developing in the womb.

Fundamentals of Eating Right

A person must ensure that their meal is balanced. A balanced meal contains essential nutrients like carbohydrates, proteins, fats, vitamins, minerals, and fiber. Eating healthy does not need to be too difficult. Eating healthy is not about strict limitations, calorie deficits, staying too thin, or staying away from foods you love. It is more about feeling great and energetic, with good immunity and an improved mood.

The same is applicable in pregnancy as well. You must keep in mind the points mentioned below.

- **Prepare your own meal** – In this way, you know what is being added and what is not being added and can have the food in peace without fearing allergens, extra calorie intake, etc.
- **Make the correct shift** – When deciding to stay away from junk food, replace it with healthy options. E.g., choose grilled chicken or grilled fish instead of deep-fried chicken.
- **Read the labels** – Before consuming pre-packaged food, check the contents for hidden sugars and trans-fat, and added preservatives, chemical coloring agents, chemicals, and artificial flavoring agents.
- **Focus on how your mood is after eating** – The healthier the food eaten, the better the mood will be.
- **Drink plenty of water** – Do not wait till you feel thirsty; thirst is one of the primary symptoms of pregnancy. Keep sipping on water to avoid dehydration, as pregnant women PEE more often and drink less water.
- **Eat six to eight meals** – Have smaller meals and split them through the day.
- **Take your time to eat** – Digestion starts in the mouth. Ensure to chew the food well so that you are not having a large amount of food and you are giving time for the stomach to send signals to the brain regarding the fullness. DO NOT EAT while watching television or looking at your mobile. Include a lot of fruits and vegetables in the diet. If you are able to source organic fruits and vegetables, that would be the best.

Nutritional needs are higher for the mother and the baby during pregnancy. Increased nutrition is needed for the growth and development of the baby; the nutritional needs of the mother are higher as well, as she is preparing herself for many changes physically, mentally, and emotionally.

However, the grandmother's advice of EATING FOR TWO PEOPLE is WRONG. It would be more accurate to say you should eat 1.3 times of your needs, not twice. This old UNSCIENTIFIC food advice by the older generation is the reason we have more obese children today. Leave this calculation to the nutritionist! Ryan has worked with Anushka Sharma, the film star, and cricketer Virat Kohli's wife. The questions she asked Ryan were thought-provoking:

ANUSHKA: How much do I need to eat to remain FIT for my baby and me?

RYAN: Based on your body weight of muscle, fat, bone, and water, I will calculate the number of calories you need for your body. Then I will calculate how many calories are additionally required for your baby in that trimester of growth. Based on your Doctor's advice, we will also look at your scans and increase or decrease the calories and proteins as the weeks progress. We will not eyeball it. We will work scientifically.

ANUSHKA: Can you tell me exactly how much weight I should gain each week?

RYAN: Ideally, a max of 10–12 kg in your small-sized frame over the entire pregnancy. We should monitor about 250 gm of weight gain a week from the 2nd trimester onwards. We will guide you on eating right every four weeks. Along with your food diary, we help you understand when you overeat and how that affects your weight.

ANUSHKA: What should be my weight in the last weeks of my pregnancy?

RYAN: When a baby is born in India, the average birth weight is 2.5–3.5 kg. Mothers should put on a maximum of an additional 6–10 kg. Many gain 20–30 kg, and this is not healthy for both mother and baby.

ANUSHKA: How much time will it take to lose the weight and get back to my original figure once I deliver?

RYAN: With a carefully balanced diet and an exercise regime of 15,000 steps a day, you can lose 1 kg per week. However, understanding that a new baby is a new responsibility, attention to yourself is complex in the first six weeks post-pregnancy due to baby duties. I always advise my clients to walk with the baby in a pram or get a treadmill and walk and talk while your baby sleeps. You can start weight training post the 1st month of delivery unless there have been surgical interventions for the pregnancy. Then the Doctor will decide on the weight training program.

ANUSHKA: During the first few weeks, I have been experiencing nausea and have not been able to hold any food. Is losing weight normal in the first trimester?

RYAN: Losing weight in the 1st trimester is normal, and the desire to eat foods is limited. I will hold your hands through this period, and there will be foods that do settle once or twice a day in your gut. We will look to manage the food and calories in this period based on your comfort. If you like rice, we will design rice soup, rice noodles, or rice pancakes to eat when you feel like it. There will be some fruits or veggies that you will like and be able to hold down, and so that will be the go-to menu for the first three months as you decide with me, the nutritionist. I will request an omega-3 supplement and a good multivitamin in case of extreme nausea and low food intake.

ANUSHKA: I have cravings. Can I overeat those foods?

RYAN: If the food is not processed and does not come in a plastic bag, yes. Nature will allow you to eat more of it. However, we must assess what that food is. For example, if you love mangoes, I see no issues. However, if it is ice-creams, coffee, or bakery items, I will have my reservations due to the ill health and weight gain effect.

ANUSHKA: Any foods that are an absolute NO-NO?

RYAN: Caffeine, found in chocolates, tea, and coffee, is a strict no. It causes obesity in the next generation—also, no alcohol.

There is always confusion about WHAT TO EAT during pregnancy, HOW MUCH TO EAT, and WHEN TO EAT!

No one answer fits every mother. It is bio-individual. It is specific, and you need to plan your eating with a scientific perspective. Nutritional counseling and interventions with a dietician need to be an integral part of antenatal care. These must continue during pregnancy to reduce the risk of maternal, fetal, and neonatal complications. Eating right influences the short- and long-term health of both the mother and the baby.

Diet for Underweight and Overweight Mothers

In pregnancy, high-quality food, along with adequate macro- and micronutrient intake, is vital for the health status of the mother and the baby. There are precise recommendations for dietary intake of different types of nutrients in pregnancy. They vary in specific points according to the eating tradition and nutrition status. Nevertheless, if you are already carrying and are overweight, do not make the mistake of dieting. Instead, it would be best if you ate with your calories in perspective. "LESS SIMPLE CARBS, MORE COMPLEX CARBS". You can refer to some of our sample diet charts at www.quanutrition.com/pregnancydietcharts.

Do You Need to Eat for Two in Pregnancy?

The current epidemic of obesity has brought the concerns regarding weight into focus. Pregnancy is a time at which science and society diverge on the topic of weight. Unlike other times when women want to lose weight, they see pregnancy as an opportunity to ignore these concerns, as weight gain is encouraged during pregnancy.

Most of the time, during pregnancy, the mother is not being judged for eating more. Moreover, social norms use the phrase "Eating for Two". "Eating for Two" is not the right concept. Only an additional 300 calories are needed per day to achieve the 25- to 35-pound weight gain during pregnancy recommended for a normal woman. When social norms and medical evidence differ, it is crucial to rely on healthcare providers to tackle these issues. Pregnant women are focused on making sure they are eating enough, which is often too much.

Along with this, they avoid exercising to protect their unborn baby. We would argue that changing the social norms on pregnancy weight gain and the culture of "eating for two" is necessary. This will successfully help pregnant women understand the importance of, and ultimately achieve, guideline-adherent weight gain. Unlike obesity or tobacco use, excessive weight gain in pregnancy is not recognized to be harmful by society at large.

Role of Diet in Gestational Diabetes Mellitus

Gestational Diabetes Mellitus (GDM) is one of the common metabolic complications seen in pregnancy. GDM is a disorder involving at least three aspects of metabolism: insulin resistance, decreased insulin secretion, and increased glucose production.

It is essential to monitor glucose metabolism during pregnancy along with that of other nutrients. Studies have demonstrated the positive effects of following healthy eating habits before and during pregnancy. Research has shown that consuming an improper diet during pregnancy, such as a high-fat, low-carbohydrate, and/or low-fiber diet, or a diet with high glycemic load increases the risk of developing GDM.

Maternal dietary patterns play an essential role. A 2017 study showed that western dietary habits, high in sweets, jams, soft drinks, salty snacks, high-fat dairy, organ meat, egg, and processed foods, were associated with an increased risk of developing GDM. The latest research guidelines suggest that it is vital for pregnant women to consult a nutritionist for medical nutrition therapy. Special Medical Nutrition Therapy plays a substantial role in helping pregnant women with GDM. It enables them to attain and preserve normal blood sugar levels and healthy weight gain with essential macro- and micronutrients.

Role of Supplements in Pregnancy

The nutrient requirement is higher during periods of growth and development in pregnancy and during lactation. Due to this, the recommendation of dietary supplements during these periods has become critical. Even though these nutrient requirements can be met by consuming an appropriate quantity of food via properly balanced meals, supplements may be beneficial in certain situations.

Due to increased energy and nutritional demands during pregnancy, deficiencies worsen, which can be taken care of by including micronutrient supplementation. There are multivitamins, iron, calcium, zinc, folic acid, Vitamin A, Vitamin E, and Vitamin D supplements. Micronutrient or vitamin supplementation is essential to promote maternal and fetal nutrition, health, and well-being. This pattern needs to be continued to avoid ill health in the babies as they will be future mothers for the coming generations.

Myths And Truth About Diet in Pregnancy

Women have many misconceptions about nutrition during pregnancy. In a research study on common myths about nutrition in pregnancy, 90 percent of pregnant women gave wrong answers to the five questions that they were asked on the subject.

Some of the common myths and the reality are listed below.

MYTHS	TRUTHS
Prenatal vitamins are for women with vitamin or mineral deficiencies	Multivitamins made for pregnant women are for the well-being of both the mother and the baby. This is required for all pregnant women due to increased nutritional demands.
Eat for two as you need extra calories	It is not required to eat for two. It is enough to eat a healthy well-balanced diet, with an inclusion of 300 additional calories.
Weight gain is very important during pregnancy	This is not very true; it depends on the BMI of the mother at the time of conception. Most women gain too much weight during pregnancy, which is not very good. Keep a check on your weight even during pregnancy to avoid obesity post-delivery. I know of a person who lost weight during pregnancy and yet delivered a healthy weight baby. So, it does not count that the mother needs to put on weight during pregnancy.

Eating saffron results in a fair-skinned baby	Saffron has its benefits and medicinal properties, but consuming it in a large dosage can result in embryonic malfunction and miscarriage.

It is better to check with an expert dietician or nutritionist before consuming any food. Follow what is recommended by the healthcare experts as they know what they are doing.

Good Dietary Sources

A healthy diet is very crucial during pregnancy. The diet must fuel the nutritional needs of pregnant women with the correct quantity and quality of food to keep the mother and the baby healthy.

Listed below are some options of healthy superfoods that can be consumed.

- **Chia Seeds** – Chia seeds are rich in omega-3 fatty acids. It is essential for fetal brain development and also helps in preventing preterm birth.
- **Lean Meat** is rich in quality proteins, iron, choline, and vitamin B. Protein is essential for the growing fetus.
- **Green Leafy Vegetables** – Rich in iron, calcium, and folic acid. All these nutrients are essential for maintaining a healthy body during pregnancy.
- **Beans and Lentils** – They are rich in protein and fiber. Fiber helps in preventing constipation when taken in the right way.
- **Berries** are rich in antioxidants. They help in scavenging free radicals and prevent cell damage.
- **Broccoli** – It is rich in fiber, calcium, and folate. It is also rich in antioxidants. It is a rich source of vitamin C, and therefore helps better in the absorption of iron when taken along with iron-rich foods.
- **Egg** – It is rich in quality protein and contains all the essential amino acids. It is a perfect superfood for muscle development and growth in the baby.

- **Fruits** are rich in vitamins and antioxidants. They help in improving overall health and well-being. **Sweet potato** is rich in fiber and vitamin A. It helps in keeping the energy levels up and prevents tiredness.
- **Whole grains** are rich in fiber, vitamins, and minerals. They help in maintaining a healthy weight during pregnancy and are also rich in vitamins and minerals.
- **Pumpkin seeds** are a nutrient-dense option to snack on. They help improve muscle health and play a role in changes that happen post-pregnancy to get back in shape.
- **Figs** – They are rich in fiber and are an excellent non-dairy source of calcium. **Peas** are rich in folic acid, which is a vital nutrient required by the mother and the baby. Peas help improve folic acid levels.
- **Yogurt** – Rich in probiotics (good microorganisms), which help in improving gut health; they also help in better absorption of nutrients.
- Probiotics help in preventing the baby from getting eczema or other allergies in the long run.

It is necessary to consume superfoods to address any pregnancy symptoms to have a happy and safe pregnancy.

Supplements in Pregnancy Based on Scientific Background

With pregnancy, an increased need for certain nutrients is felt. During pregnancy, mothers focus on their diet to improve their own health and the future health of the fetus. Recommendations are given for pregnant women based on their requirements. Nutritionists, Dieticians, Physicians, and other healthcare providers play an essential role and offer accurate and evidence-based supplement information to expectant mothers. These supplements need not be taken for a long time. It is only for individuals who are at risk.

Omega-3 fatty acid supplements are required for pregnant mothers as most of them cannot meet the daily requirement with diet alone. This is because most of the omega fatty acids are sourced from seafood, and there are restrictions on the consumption of seafood by pregnant women.

Omega-3 fatty acids play a vital role in fetal neurodevelopment, and are necessary during the gestation period for the baby to be born with a healthy birth weight. A study was conducted on pregnant women, where they were divided into three sub-groups. The first group of women received fish oil supplements, the second group received olive oil supplements, and the third did not receive either of these. The results were thought-provoking.

Women who had consumed fish oil delivered babies who weighed 107 gm more than the babies of the women who had consumed olive oil. The second group of women had babies who weighed 43 gm more than the babies of the women who did not consume fish oil or olive oil.

You can read about this study at the link given below.
https://www.ncbi.nlm.nih.gov/pmc/articles/ PMC2621042/.

Iron is one of the common supplements that is usually prescribed for any pregnant woman. There has been much research regarding iron supplementation: the effects of supplementation with 60 mg, 50 mg, and 30 mg elemental iron have been studied.

Women who received supplementary iron during pregnancy showed a reduced risk of developing anemia compared to the risk shown by women who did not consume supplementary iron. A difference of 47 percent was demonstrated between the anemic state of those who received iron supplements and those who had not. Iron supplemented women also had a 12 percent reduced risk of delivering low-birth-weight babies.

Vitamin D supplementation during pregnancy can be administered once the mother has checked her vitamin D levels and has found it deficient. Various studies have been conducted in South Asia, Bangladesh, and India on vitamin D supplementation in pregnancy. Some of these studies were on women who were given vitamin D supplementation till the end of their pregnancy.

In contrast, the rest of the studies were conducted on women who were given the supplementation only for a shorter period, according to their requirements. Results showed that vitamin D supplements helped in decreasing the risk of preterm birth by 36 percent. However, it did not affect the risk of having a C-section delivery or the serum calcium levels; instead, it increased the vitamin D concentrations in the mothers.

You can visit the link below to know more about this study.
https://www.ncbi.nlm.nih.gov/pmc/articles/PMC70/ #B77-nutrients-12-00491

Folic acid is one of the essential supplements required for DNA replication, enzymatic reactions in amino acid synthesis, and vitamin metabolism. Folic acid demand is heightened during pregnancy as it is necessary for the growth and development of the baby. A folate deficiency can lead to abnormalities in both the mother and the baby. Folic acid supplements help in protecting from fetal structural abnormalities like neural tube disorders and congenital heart defects. Recent studies have found that it also helps in preventing preterm birth.

Please read the article given in the link below for further information.
www.ncbi.nlm.nih.gov/pmc/articles/ PMC3218540/

Remember to eat in moderation. Do not take all the advice of the elders. Some of it is slowly turning out to be very unscientific. Turn to your Doctor for advice. Ask for a nutritionist or dietician to help you plan your eating as you carry your baby. Any advice I have given is generic. Do not self-prescribe your diet or your supplements from the Internet or other articles. Ryan Fernando has given a thought-provoking message on what to eat during pregnancy. Like food, another major concept needed to be discussed here is the right type of physical exercise needed during pregnancy. In the next chapter, we will discuss fitness during pregnancy.

8

FITNESS DURING PREGNANCY

Do you think that pregnancy is a time for complete physical rest? If so, then you are wrong. Pregnancy does not force you to take rest throughout your journey. You need a good amount of exercise during this phase for a safe and easy delivery. I have encountered many women who have asked me about exercises and the duration of activities they could take up during pregnancy.

Being a Radiologist, I have some limitations in giving advice on this topic. My wife too asked me the same question during her pregnancy, and I was speechless as I did not have an answer. I informed her that I was not qualified to give any advice on that subject.

She teased me and asked me if I was a real Doctor. I have seen a similar attitude in many women who pose the same question to me. Now, I have the answer for all who wish to know about exercise in pregnancy.

Physio Meghna Dave will provide the answers. Let us hear what she has to say about exercise in pregnancy: You are nurturing a new life, a new being. There is a lot of excitement, happiness, and preparedness. A lot is happening inside the body as your hormones change. As your baby grows in size, your posture changes.

So does the health of your bones, muscles, and joints. Many women are unaware of the changes that happen to their body during this phase.

Your musculoskeletal system needs that extra strength to cope up with all the changes happening in the body. Moreover, one such thing that your body needs is physical exercise.

I am sure you must have heard of antenatal exercises, but have you ever wondered WHY you need these EXERCISES? Well, I hope some of these reasons might convince you to choose to exercise for a healthy pregnancy: Mild-to-moderate–intensity exercises are beneficial for both the mother and the fetus in low-risk pregnancies with the necessary modifications.

You are more prone to gain excessive weight during pregnancy. The potential risk of excessive weight gain is the higher risk of developing GDM or hypertension, or undergoing a C-section delivery. Some of the benefits of exercise during pregnancy are as listed:

- Exercise helps you maintain cardiovascular and respiratory fitness.
- It keeps you more relaxed and helps you cope with the emotional changes that you experience during pregnancy.
- Exercises also develop your baby's brain, and keeps the baby more interested and alert to the surroundings.
- No less importantly, you will be able to lose your weight post-pregnancy quickly.

Is Exercising the Right Thing for You?

Well, there are some conditions and situations when you should avoid exercise. However, it is always better to discuss with your Gynecologist whether you are fit for physical activities. One of my friends mentioned a pregnant woman who came for regular exercise sessions at his clinic. She attended the sessions till her fifth month and was absent from then onwards. She contacted the patient's husband, whose mobile number was in the register, to learn the reason for her absence. Her husband mentioned that his wife did not need to exercise anymore as she had already delivered her baby. My friend did not understand what he meant and decided to inquire about this case from another client who had come along with her.

He was shocked to learn that the woman had suffered a miscarriage, and she had been diagnosed to have an incompetent cervix from the very beginning of her pregnancy. She was restricted from doing any physical labor; however, she ignored this advice and visited the clinic because she wanted to have a normal vaginal delivery rather than a C-section delivery.

After narrating this incident, my friend advised me that, when pregnant women come for a session, I should always cross-check about their medical conditions with their bystanders and their Doctors, to avoid such accidents. You should avoid exercises if you have the following medical conditions:

1. Ruptured membranes
2. History of premature labor in a previous pregnancy
3. Unexplained prolonged vaginal bleeding
4. Low placental location
5. Pre-eclampsia
6. Incompetent cervix (short cervix)
7. Fetus growth restriction (FGR)
8. High-order multiple pregnancy (e.g., triplets, quadruplets)
9. Uncontrolled Type I Diabetes
10. Uncontrolled hypertension
11. Uncontrolled thyroid disease
12. Severe heart, lung, or systemic disorders

Likewise, if you belong to any of the following categories, you should be a little careful while exercising.

i) Recurrent pregnancy loss
ii) Gestational hypertension (high BP)
iii) A history of spontaneous preterm birth
iv) Mild-to-moderate cardiovascular or respiratory disease
v) Symptomatic anemia
vi) Malnutrition
vii) Eating disorder
viii) Twin pregnancy after the 28th week

By now, you must be thinking, WHAT kind of exercises can I do during pregnancy, right? There are many exercise formats that you can adopt during Pregnancy. Your choice of exercise format will depend on these factors:

i) What you enjoy doing?
ii) What is suitable for your body type?
iii) What is feasible for you?
iv) What is necessary for you?

If you are a regular person, as far as exercise is concerned, you should continue exercising to maintain your fitness level rather than trying to reach your peak performance during pregnancy. So here are the exercise formats that you can take up during your pregnancy journey.

Let us analyze them one by one.

- **Aerobic exercises**: E.g., ZUMBA, treadmill, brisk walking, swimming
- **Cycling**: A low-intensity exercise
- **Pilates**: Pilates improves balance, strength and flexibility, and posture
- **Running**: But only if you were a runner before becoming pregnant
- **Strength training**: Basically, gym-based exercises
- **Yoga**: It not only helps in improving flexibility, but also helps in improving wellness

Meet your Doctor or a Physiotherapist, take their suggestions, and start the exercise format based on their advice. Physio Meghna Dave has briefed you with enough inputs on the benefits of exercise, who shouldn't be exercising and also, the different formats of exercises during pregnancy. There is an online platform named "Pregawell" that might help you stay fit during your pregnancy journey. Another important area that needs to be discussed concerning exercise in pregnancy is Yoga. Let us discuss that in the next chapter.

9

PRENATAL YOGA

My friend and a famous prenatal yoga therapist named Priya Nair, the co-founder of "Pregawell," has offered this chapter that will aid you in learning some useful tips about practicing yoga during pregnancy. The word 'yoga' comes from a Sanskrit word that means "to unite". While doing yoga, your individual self or individual consciousness unites with the universal consciousness. That is why yoga is recommended during pregnancy, as it unites your individual self and your baby's self with the universal consciousness.

I have seen many women commenting about yoga and the significance of it during pregnancy. Out of curiosity, I asked a patient to define the type of yoga practiced during pregnancy. She looked at me and mentioned that the yoga she has been practicing throughout her life is what she practices during pregnancy.

I got a bit confused on hearing it, so I decided to study more about prenatal yoga. Prenatal yoga is very gentle when compared to regular yoga. It is right to say that prenatal yoga has great importance in elevating the health of the mother and the child. You might not be able to practice many of the postures that you were practicing before getting pregnant, as the growing tummy might hinder it. It is essential to pick up yoga techniques that will suit your physical, mental, and emotional capacities at this time.

It is also helpful in preparing the mother to accept her new responsibilities and connect with the baby. Let us check some of the benefits of undertaking prenatal yoga.

They include the following:
- Enhances strength, flexibility, and endurance
- Relieves back pain and sciatica
- Removes stress and anxiety
- Elevates sleep
- Removes swelling and inflammation around the joints
- Helps in digestion

The list goes on, and it is challenging to pinpoint all the benefits of prenatal yoga. Are you aware of the postural changes that happen during pregnancy? You might know that the abdomen enlarges along with the growth of the child. However, this growing abdomen paves the way to several other changes in body posture. Let us analyze them one by one.

- All spinal curvatures are increased. Our spine has three major curvatures: cervical lordosis, present in the neck portion; thoracic kyphosis, present in the back portion of the chest; and lumbar lordosis, present in the lumbar region.
- With the growing girth of the abdomen, the curvatures bend to accommodate the baby within the womb. The head shifts forward, and the chin gets tucked in. As the baby grows, to maintain the balance of the body with the growing abdomen, our chin automatically tucks in. Many of you might be unaware of these changes. Breasts become enlarged and heavy, which is very uncomfortable as they are constrained by the underlying ribcage. Above all, the center of gravity shifts forward.

All these postural changes lead to muscular imbalances. Prenatal yoga helps in managing all these postural and muscular changes happening during pregnancy. Before enrolling yourself for a prenatal yoga session, it is essential to get clearance from your Doctor. You should not undertake prenatal yoga if you have pregnancy issues or belong to a high-risk pregnancy category mentioned in the previous chapter.

Hence, you should ask permission from your Obstetrician before joining prenatal yoga sessions. Then it is vital to talk to your yoga instructor regarding your medical conditions and what you expect from prenatal yoga. You might not practice yoga as before; hence, practice what you feel is right. Take your time to practice the postures slowly so that your body gets enough time to get used to these techniques along with the rapid changes happening to your body.

During this time, it is essential to use props and make necessary modifications to the postures. It is advisable to include techniques that act as 'hip openers' and 'pelvic strengtheners' during the practice. As mentioned earlier, your center of gravity changes; hence, practice the techniques slowly to avoid danger.

Safe Yoga Poses During Pregnancy

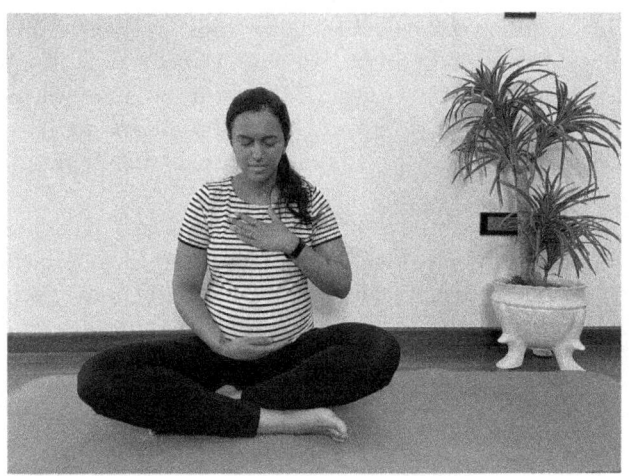

Breathing Yoga Pose

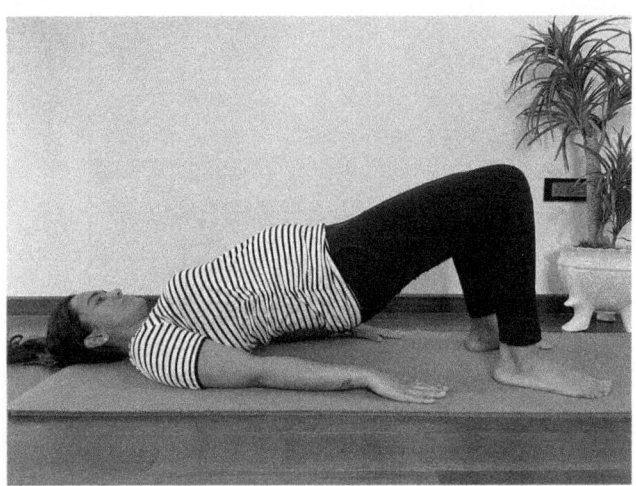

Bridge Pose- Setu Bandhasana

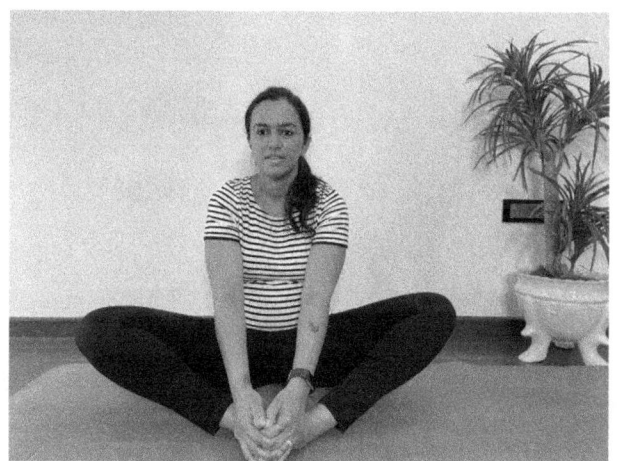
Butterfly Pose - Baddhakonasana

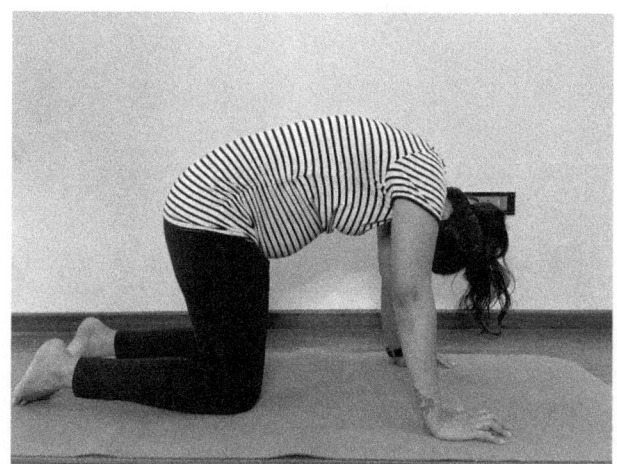
Camel Stretch - Marjaryasana

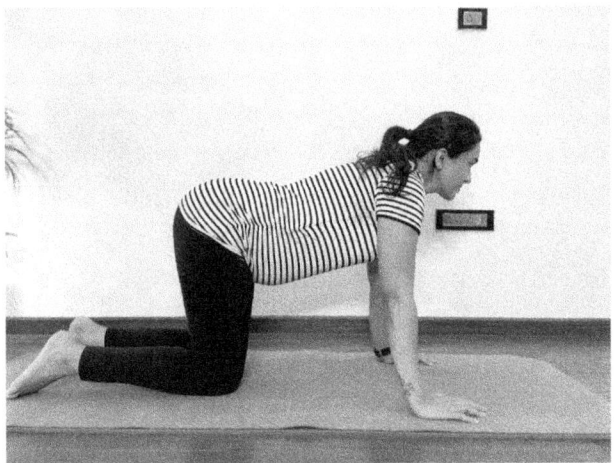

Cat Stretch - Marjaryasana

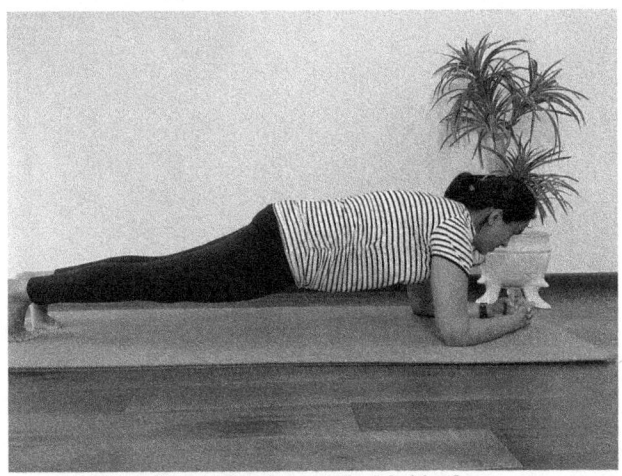

Elbow Plank - Makara Adho Mukha Svanasana

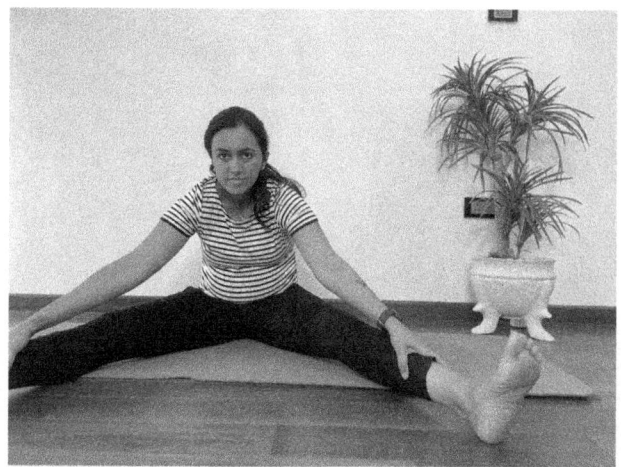
Wide-Legged Seated Forward Bend - Upavistha Konasana

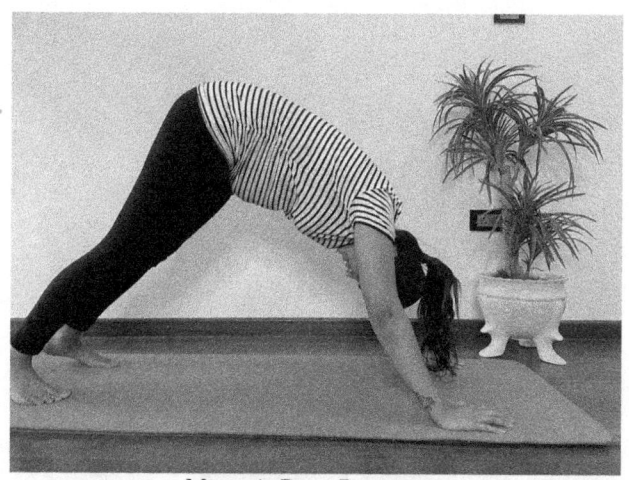
Mountain Pose - Parvatasana

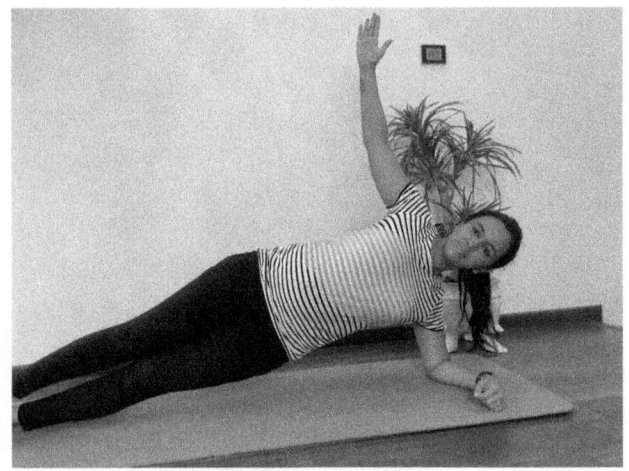

Side Elbow Plank - Vasisth Asana

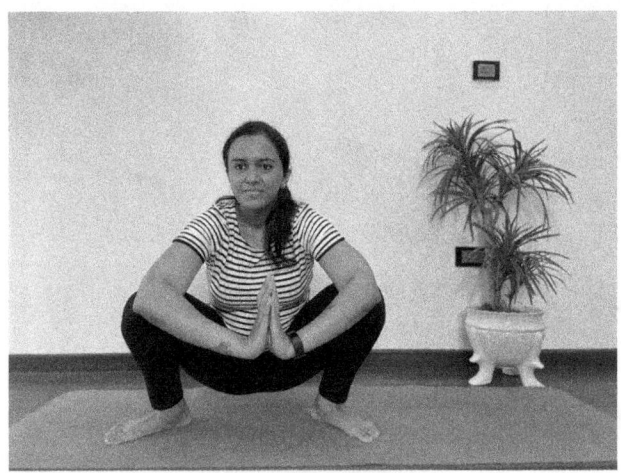

Garland Pose - Malasana

In case you notice symptoms such as vaginal bleeding, lasting dizziness, increasing shortness of breath, chest pain, calf pain or swelling, uterine contractions, decreased baby movements, and leaking from the vagina, it is imperative to mention the issue to your Obstetrician.

Never try to continue your yoga practice along with these symptoms. There are many things you should not do while doing prenatal yoga. Never practice yoga on an empty stomach as it might affect the mother as well as the baby.

With an empty stomach, the mother will be vulnerable to muscle cramps and pains. You should also make sure to practice low-intensity yoga. Likewise, forward bends in standing posture should be avoided as you might lose your balance while doing so.

Another essential factor you ought to understand about prenatal yoga is that you should change the type of yoga techniques you practice as the pregnancy progresses. Usually, in the first trimester, which is considered a delicate period, Doctors advise their patients to avoid exercises, including yoga. Even though the Doctors are against the norm of yoga practice during this phase, it is safe to practice it. Let us look into the different techniques you could take up during this phase.

Asanas: Asanas help in the relaxation of the muscles, nerves, and joints. They also aid in creating a positive feel and increase flexibility, thereby promoting the free flow of energy throughout the body. Asanas are gentle yoga techniques that focus on strengthening the body and relaxing it to accept the new changes.

In the first trimester, you could take up simple forward bends, backward bends, and twists. However, as the pregnancy progresses, these are not advisable.

Pranayama: Pranayama is very helpful in improving sleep, which is an essential ingredient for a healthy pregnancy. It also helps in enhancing mindfulness and cognitive performance.

Meditation: Meditation helps you connect with the universe, and hence it is the preferred yoga during pregnancy. It aids in acquiring positive affirmations. However, when you enter the second trimester, these techniques should be done with modifications and with the help of props and a companion.

Just like the second trimester, extra care has to be taken while undertaking yoga during the post-pregnancy period. Postnatal yoga is also essential, just like prenatal yoga. If you had a normal delivery, you could start gentle yoga once you complete 45 days. However, in the case of a C-section delivery, it is advisable to restart yoga after three months. I hope you have got some ideas on the benefits of prenatal yoga during pregnancy.

Similar to exercise, another major component needed for a comfortable pregnancy journey is adequate rest and a good sleeping posture. As your body is busy preparing you for the "big day", it always paves the way for fatigue. Hence, a good amount of rest is needed for you, which can be enhanced by the comfortable sleeping posture that you have discovered for yourself. Let us discuss rest and sleeping posture in the next chapter.

10

RESTING AND SLEEPING POSTURE

Being pregnant by itself is a tiring and stressful condition. One of the significant issues faced by every pregnant woman is getting a full night's composed sleep, which is felt throughout the nine months of pregnancy. Good sleep is very much necessary for the baby's growth and the well-being of the mother.

During the early days of the pregnancy, you may experience excessive sleepiness due to tiredness from nausea and vomiting. The sleep problem settles down as you complete three months of pregnancy.

The problem arises again as the pregnancy advances. My wife had similar issues with sleep after her eighth month due to the baby's kicks and her growing tummy. The growing baby bump will pose difficulty for you to sleep or rest on your back or the tummy (face down). Your sleep is affected by the posture you are not naturally accustomed to.

You will experience back pain while sleeping on your back for an extended period. Sleeping on your back or the right side for a longer time will compress the large blood vessels, mainly the inferior vena cava. The compressed blood vessels can cause poor circulation in the legs, resulting in ankle and foot swelling.

There will also be insufficient blood supply to the placenta, resulting in inadequate oxygen and nutrient supply to the baby.

One of the most troubling questions in pregnancy is the proper sleeping posture. One day a pregnant woman came for her 3 D scan and argued with one of my colleagues. As the ultrasound came out, I decided to intervene to find a solution to the argument.

She was not ready to lie down on her back for the scan as her Doctor had advised her not to lie down in that posture. The idea she raised was something that disturbed all the waiting pregnant ladies. I had to convince the lady that lying down was alright as long as she was comfortable in that posture.

Later, I obtained the contact details of her Obstetrician for a consultation. The Obstetrician was helpless. The patient had complained about severe back pain, and the Obstetrician had advised her to lie down on her side to avoid further pain. The Doctor had only suggested a good sleeping posture for her, which she mistook as the only posture to be used while lying down.

I have heard many women complaining about their inability to find a proper resting posture, which in turn results in severe back pain and pelvic pain. It is advised to sleep on your side. Either side is acceptable; however, sleeping on the left side is preferred since it does not compress the blood vessels.

Keeping your knees bent and placing a pillow between the thighs or legs will provide more comfort. If you find yourself sleeping on your back for a long time, do not feel guilty. Just roll back onto your side and try to fall asleep. You may choose to rest on a sofa, chair, or recliner with legs elevated on a soft pillow during the daytime. Remember to take a small nap during the day if you have the luxury of time. You can use the pregnancy pillow or an extra regular pillow to support your tummy. Some common reasons for disturbed sleep and tips to overcome the problem are as follows:

1. **Anxiety of unknown cause or the fear of delivery:**
   Thinking about the responsibilities of becoming a mother is a stressful condition for many women. Relax, and talk to your husband and family members. You can also share your concerns with your Doctor. Sometimes a small dose of anxiety-relieving medicine will help reduce the stress. I recall meeting Arundhati, a pregnant woman who used to come for an ultrasound scan regularly.

She was suffering from anxiety. Her anxiety had run amok, causing her to imagine non-existing complications. So, she took frequent ultrasound scans to ensure the baby was fine. After talking with her, I realized that she was anxious about the baby. Many women like Arundhati are anxious about the well-being of the baby they are carrying. I informed the case to her Obstetrician, who prescribed her medications.

2. **Leg cramps can be a reason for disturbed sleep:**
   The calf muscle in some individuals can contract excessively due to a deficiency of certain minerals like calcium and magnesium. Multivitamin supplements may be beneficial to overcome leg cramps. Alternatively, you can apply pain-relieving oils or cream over the calf muscles before you go to bed.
   A friend of mine named Siddharth told me that he was not getting enough sleep at night as his wife was pregnant. This statement confused me. He narrated that his wife woke up at midnight due to leg cramps, after which he could not sleep properly.
   I suggested that he apply some pain-relieving oils on his wife's legs before she went to sleep. One week later, I got a call from him. He thanked me for suggesting the medicine as it was helpful for both of them.

3. **Making frequent trips to the restroom can interrupt sleep:**
   The urinary bladder presses on the uterus as the pregnancy grows, resulting in frequent urination. Try emptying the bladder before going to bed to avoid frequent visits to the toilet at night.

4. **Excessive baby movements may be a reason for sleep interruption:**
   My cousin once mentioned that while she was pregnant with her daughter, the baby was more active during the night. She used to get strong kicks at night, which was a significant hurdle for her peaceful sleep. Even after the delivery, the baby continued this sleeping pattern for the first three months.

5. **Heartburn:**
   The gastric juices can irritate the food pipe and throat. The condition causes a burning sensation in the chest. This can be prevented to a large extent by avoiding late dinners.
   Try to finish eating your dinner at least two hours before bedtime. Consume any fruits or light desserts before going to bed. Even if you feel hungry at night, try to consume fruits, rather than snacks.

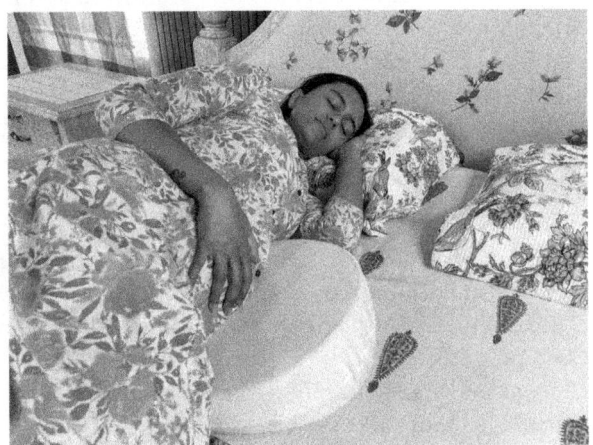

Pregnancy Pillow to support the tummy

Tips to Improve the Quality of Your Sleep

Schedule a regular sleep time. Your daytime nap should be very short so that you get adequate sleep at night. Create a good sleeping environment. Stay away from the television and mobile before going to bed. Read good books before sleeping, if you have the habit of reading. Light exercise before bedtime will help you get a sound sleep. Avoid spicy food and finish eating two to three hours before going to bed. Gentle oil massage to the calf muscles will help relieve muscle cramps. Keep your foot in warm water for 10 minutes before going to bed. Drinking hot milk will also aid in getting a sound sleep.

I hope these pointers will be helpful for you, especially during your pregnancy journey. Another major doubt that pregnant couples often raise concerns the mode of work and travel they could take up during their pregnancy journey. In the next chapter, let us analyze the work and travel modes a pregnant woman could take up.

11

WORK AND TRAVEL DURING PREGNANCY

Many women have doubts regarding work and travel during pregnancy. We have here Dr. Jyoti Kala, who will provide her insights on this topic from her experience as an Obstetrician in Bangalore. She mentioned that the most common questions asked by pregnant couples are related to work and travel during pregnancy. If you have a normal and low-risk pregnancy, you can continue to work throughout your pregnancy interval. Some basic alterations to your work schedule would help you stay comfortable at the workplace without compromising your health or the health of your baby. Many women continue to work till the end of the ninth month of pregnancy. I remember meeting Adwaitha, a 23-year-old woman, who continued to work till a week before her estimated due date. However, she delivered the baby the very next day. With a low-risk pregnancy, it is alright to continue your work till the labor pain begins. The following steps will help you in easing out the discomforts you may experience during your work time.

- Take frequent breaks, about every half hour. Get up from your seat and walk around the room. Stretch your back and exercise your shoulder and neck muscles to avoid strain.

- Elevate your feet while sitting by placing a short stool below your feet. This helps to reduce fluid retention in the lower limbs and prevents swelling of the feet.
- Wear comfortable clothing and footwear.
- Drink plenty of fluids (around 2.5 L per day) and avoid holding urine for extended intervals.
- Eat at regular intervals and do not skip meals.
- If you get tired during work, take a short break to rejuvenate.
- If work becomes too stressful, consider reducing your workplace responsibilities or taking a break from work till required.

These simple measures can go a long way in helping you continue and enjoy your work during pregnancy.

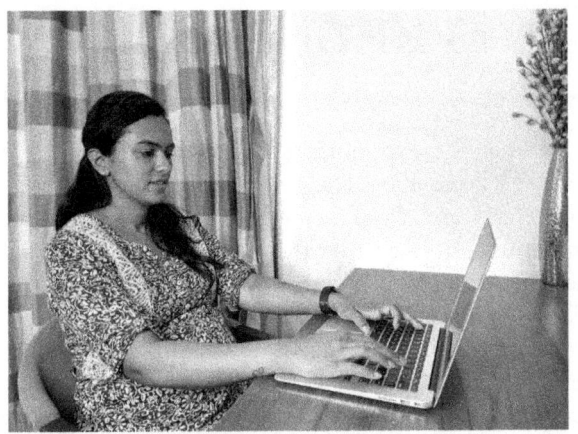

Work during pregnancy

Travel During Pregnancy

Most women are anxious regarding travel during pregnancy. Traveling before the 12th week might be more troublesome when early pregnancy symptoms like nausea and vomiting are still bothering you. The risk of bleeding or miscarriage is also higher in the first trimester. Likewise, as pregnancy proceeds beyond 28 weeks, travel might become physically more uncomfortable with your growing tummy.

So, the mid-pregnancy interval between 14 and 28 weeks is considered the most comfortable time to travel. My senior mentioned a patient named Ankitha, who came with her bucket list during her third-month pregnancy check-up. He was shocked to see "visit Ladakh in the fourth month" among the entries and enquired about the list.

Ankitha mentioned that her husband was a long-distance bike rider, and as she was safe from the 14th week to the 28th week, they had decided to travel to Ladakh or somewhere closer on their bike. This dream of Ankitha's was troubling, and the Doctor immediately cut the entry from the list and stated the risk factors associated with traveling on a bike for such a long distance.

After narrating this incident, he commented, "Many patients might approach you with their bucket list. Make sure to put enough water in the bucket so that the list becomes invisible." Indirectly, he mentioned never to approve such dangerous and tiresome dreams and fancies of pregnant women.

Long-distance travel is not recommended beyond 36 weeks, as the risk of going into labor *en route* becomes high. On my best friend's wedding eve, I was called to the hospital amidst my leave. As my senior was also on holiday, I was asked to attend an emergency placental abruption case. I barely remember her name as she was not our patient.

The pregnant woman was staying in Kodur, and the family was traveling to Kerala, her hometown, as her due date was approaching. She was 37 weeks pregnant, and her Obstetrician had actually restricted her from traveling in the car as her due date was near.

On the way, her water broke, and she started experiencing vaginal bleeding. As normal delivery was not an option, the doctor immediately did a C-section and took the baby out. This incident is proof that even car journeys during the last phase of pregnancy should not be allowed. She was fortunate enough to be traveling through Bangalore at that time.

The story would have had a different ending if they were stranded in some rural area when the water broke. Travel by road, train, or flight is considered safe in the mid-pregnancy period; however, it is advisable to avoid travel during the later phases of pregnancy. You can take certain precautions to ensure that you have a comfortable journey.

- Keep yourself well hydrated and take regular bathroom breaks. Avoid sitting beyond four hours to prevent the risk of clots forming in the blood vessels of the legs (deep vein thrombosis).
- You can get up and walk every four hours in case of a flight journey or stop your car to stretch and walk.
- The seat belt should be worn below your tummy bulge (across your hip bones) and not over your tummy.
- Avoid long-distance travel if you develop any concerns before your trip, like abdomen pain, watery or blood-stained discharge, or increased lower backache. In such cases, please consult your Gynecologist or the nearest hospital immediately.
- Make sure to relax throughout the journey.

Additional Information on Air Travel in Pregnancy Sourced from the Official Site of DGCA:

The rules are slightly different for different airlines. It is good to contact the airline operator or refer to the airline website for clarifications. General pointers are discussed for air travel in this section. An expectant mother in good health can take up an air trip till the 32nd week of pregnancy. In cases where the pregnancy has advanced beyond 32 weeks, and a normal delivery is anticipated, the expectant mother will be allowed to travel up to and including the 36th week of pregnancy. In other words, she can travel up to at least four weeks before the expected delivery date. A medical certificate from the attending Obstetrician must be obtained stating that she is fit to travel. If there is an interval of more than one month between the booking and departure dates, an additional certificate should be obtained, dated not more than three days before departure. Women with multiple and complicated pregnancies will not be allowed to fly after 32 weeks in certain cases:

- Multiple pregnancy, which refers to twins, triplets, etc., as the mother-to-be needs more care.
- Complicated pregnancy, which refers to cases where on previous occasions, a mother has experienced complicated and challenging delivery.

In case of pregnancy beyond 35 weeks, the passenger may be accepted for transportation only on urgent or compassionate grounds; they need to fill in the medical information form (MEDIF) and they will be permitted to fly under the authority of The Executive Director - Medical Services.

Newborn Baby

Sometimes, newborn babies are also made to travel by air in emergencies. Some critical factors to note while planning for such a journey are as follows:
- The infant should be 14 days old before air travel.
- Exceptionally, for life-saving treatment for the newborn, the mother and baby can be accepted for travel, before 14 days, with medical certificates from the Obstetrician and a Pediatrician. These passengers have to be accompanied by a Doctor. In such cases, an indemnity has to be obtained from the passenger, as in the case of MEDA passengers. SOURCE: AIR INDIA.

In the next chapter, let us discuss the changes that occur to your skin once you start your pregnancy journey.

12

SKINCARE DURING PREGNANCY

I recall meeting a nine-month pregnant woman who came for her late month scan. The skin on her abdomen had extensive scars as if she had been scratched by a tiger. When questioned about it by our scan assistant who accompanied her, she mentioned that she experienced severe itching in the skin on the abdomen throughout her pregnancy. She resorted to scratching to relieve the itching and this resulted in scarring.

I was reminded of this incident when my wife got pregnant. When we received the good news, I informed her of this incident and we decided to consult a Dermatologist. Without much doubt, we decided to meet Dr. Sapna Revankar, who has given significant inputs into the skincare techniques that could be used during pregnancy.

When I started writing this book, I thought of including a chapter on skincare as it is important. Skincare is something many women ignore during pregnancy as they are mainly occupied with the baby's health.

Let me dive straight into the different skin conditions during pregnancy. Common skin conditions can be separated into three categories during pregnancy:

1. Hormone-related skin conditions,
2. Pre-existing skin conditions, and
3. Pregnancy-specific skin conditions.

During pregnancy, hormone changes may cause skin problems, such as Striae gravidarum (stretch marks), Hyper-pigmentation, and hair and nail changes. Pre-existing skin conditions such as atopic dermatitis, psoriasis, and fungal infections may change during pregnancy. There are chances that these conditions may flare-up during pregnancy.

Let us analyze a few common skin conditions.

Striae Gravidarum (Stretch Marks):

This condition starts to develop by the third trimester of pregnancy. Striae appear as pink/purple lines or bands on the abdomen, buttocks, breasts, thighs, or arms. The cause of striae could be either excessive stretching of the skin or the action of hormonal factors like adrenocortical steroids, estrogen, and relaxin on the skin's elastic fibers.

One of my friends once referred to a patient who had long, red-colored stretch marks on her body. As she experienced severe itching when the skin stretched during pregnancy, she scratched them to get relief from the discomfort.

This caused intense and very prominent marks. Creams, emollients, and oils (e.g., vitamin E cream, cocoa butter) can be used to hydrate the skin. Evidence suggests that topical treatments may help reduce striae.

Most striae fade to pale or flesh-colored lines and shrink after delivery, although they usually do not disappear completely. Laser and PRP procedures are other treatment options.

Chloasma:

During pregnancy, the skin color changes due to pigmentation. The breast areola, armpits, and genitals are the most commonly affected areas. Chloasma is also called melasma when it occurs on the face. In case of severe Chloasma, topical applications and depigmenting procedures can be undertaken.

Acne:

Facial acne (pimples) tends to get worse during pregnancy. The pregnancy hormones cause increased secretion of the oil glands, which ultimately results in a breakout. Hence, clean your face with a mild cleanser in the morning and evening. Use non-comedogenic skincare products. There are various treatments available that are safe to use during pregnancy.

Cholestasis of Pregnancy:

An itchy skin should not be ignored in pregnancy. Cholestasis of pregnancy is a liver condition that results from high amounts of pregnancy hormones affecting the normal flow of bile. This condition occurs in the third trimester and can cause severe itching over the whole body. It can be worse on the palms and soles of the feet and causes patients to feel miserable and unable to sleep. A blood test can verify if you have cholestasis during pregnancy. Oral medication is usually provided to treat the condition. It subsides post-delivery.

Other rare skin conditions include Pruritic urticarial papules, Plaques, Prurigo, Pemphigoid gestationis, and Impetigo herpetiformis. All these rare skin conditions require professional advice. Most of these troublesome skin conditions resolve after pregnancy. However, never consume any medicine without getting a proper consultation and prescription from the Dermatologist. In the next chapter, let us learn about the mental health that is important in your pregnancy journey.

13

MENTAL HEALTH IN PREGNANCY

Pregnancy brings about significant changes in the life of every woman. All changes and discomforts experienced during and after pregnancy need close monitoring. Mental disorders such as depression, anxiety, and psychological distress are common during pregnancy.

In this chapter, I introduce to you a Psychiatrist and a close acquaintance of mine, Dr. Sharanabasavaraj Devaramani, who will share his insights on mental health in pregnancy. Many mental health–related conditions during pregnancy are triggered by personal experiences, family history of psychiatric illness, substance abuse, sexual, physical, or emotional abuse, and/or ongoing adverse life events. While pursuing my masters in psychiatry, I learned about a woman named Annie from one of my professors. She was my professor's great aunt, who committed suicide while she was pregnant. He narrated this incident to us to inform us about the psychological condition of women during pregnancy. Annie belonged to a family with a history of bipolar affective disorder. Her uncle had bipolar affective disorder; the treatment for this condition was not available back then. Hence, he was termed a mad person and put in the sanatorium as a part of the treatment.

Annie was happily married off to Avarachan, a wealthy landowner in Kottayam. She was a government official who earned a good salary during that time. However, she was disturbed to find her father-in-law collecting her salary from the treasury without her permission.

Three months after the wedding, Avarachan got a new job and moved abroad, leaving behind his one-month pregnant wife with his father. As Avarachan's mother was not alive, Annie decided to go to her ancestral home for better care. The fact that her father-in-law was withdrawing Annie's salary was a disturbing factor for her family members too.

During her stay, her mother also criticized her for staying quiet on the matter. Disturbed by her father-in-law's actions and her mother's constant yelling, her dormant depression showed up, resulting in her suicide. After the narration, our professor posed a question: What action led to the suicide? Many answers popped up, and at last, my professor said that all the answers were correct. However, the main underlying reason was the family history of bipolar affective disorder.

In most cases, family histories are neglected. Annie's life was an excellent example of how past events, disturbing incidents, and living environment can disturb a pregnant woman's psyche. Psychological disturbances associated with pregnancy are also related to improper antenatal care. Postpartum depression is associated with low emotional involvement, negligence, and hostility toward the newborn.

I had another patient named Jyothirmayi who suffered from postpartum depression. She was reluctant to feed the baby and claimed that her husband loved the baby more than he loved her. As the family could not identify the issue, they took her to an Obstetrician, assuming she had problems in feeding the baby. While talking to the Obstetrician, she mentioned her fear, which grabbed the attention of the Doctor.

Her Doctor suggested that she consult a Psychiatrist. Jyothirmayi was a working woman and had been with her husband's parents throughout the pregnancy as her office was close to their house. During counselling, she mentioned that she did not get enough attention from her husband's parents. Her sister-in-law was also pregnant, and her in-laws were more concerned about their daughter than about their daughter-in-law.

This was only her misconception, which I realized after speaking with her in-laws. I informed her parents and asked them to come and stay with her. This is not an isolated case; I have encountered several instances where the pregnant woman experiences such misconceptions and hallucinations

Mental Issues During Pregnancy

Prevalence of antenatal depression or anxiety ranges from 8%–30% during pregnancy. The strongest predictors for antenatal depressive symptoms are a history of depression, stressful life events experienced in the year before pregnancy, and depressive symptoms during pregnancy.

Geetika was a patient who had antenatal depression. She had a miscarriage six months before the successful pregnancy. As she was obese, her Doctor advised her to take a good amount of rest during her first pregnancy. However, due to a family emergency, she travelled to her native village near Chandigarh from Bangalore. The air travel was fine; however, the subsequent road journey by car led to a miscarriage. She was disheartened at that time and nearly killed herself by consuming too many medicines.

When it came to her husband's notice, she was immediately taken to a hospital and was saved. The junior Doctor, who attended to her case, suggested a second pregnancy to relieve her depressive mood. However, this led to further issues as she started developing depression during the second pregnancy, which happened five months after the incident.

Geetika's husband and parents brought her to me for advice, and I prescribed her medications that could be used during pregnancy. Within no time, she was back on her feet; she was on medication for one more year. Once she became stable, I started tapering the medication, and within one year, she had completely stopped taking it. Restricted social activities and miscarriage add to the stress factors in pregnancy. In some developing countries, being single, having multiple partners, having a previous history of stillbirth, and a perceived lack of social support were associated with depression. Furthermore, the quality of the marital relationship, adequate social support, and self-confidence protected women from distress. In one of our class lectures, our professor mentioned Radhika, who had been taking medication for depression even before her marriage.

When she became pregnant, her husband and the other family members were worried about the consequences of hormones on her mental health. Radhika was my professor's patient, and they informed him about her pregnancy. Throughout her pregnancy, her parents and husband have been with her and supported her in every manner. More than her parent's support, the support offered by her husband helped her make it through the pregnancy journey without any distress or harm. The more support and comfort your partner offers, the happier and more content you will be throughout your pregnancy.

Mental Issues During the Postnatal Phase:

Around 12%–16% of women experience postpartum depression, which is called postpartum blues. Roma, a 20-year-old mother, was suffering from postpartum depression as her astrologer predicted a son instead of a daughter. She gave birth to a daughter, a depressive factor for her, as her in-laws also wished for a grandson. It took four months for her to come out of this depressive element and be happy with the baby that God had blessed her with. I always advise patients to ignore such predictions.

To convince Roma, I narrated real-life incidents where such predictions turned out to be incorrect. It is a request to all pregnant women out there: Never go with such predictions as it might later create issues with your relationship with your child. Studies have shown that educated mothers manifested fewer mental disorders, low stress levels, and also good marital relations. Such women are less likely to exhibit mental health problems. Depressed mothers had lower birth weight babies, and the rate of spontaneous preterm birth was significantly higher among women with high depression scores.

One of the best ways to get rid of postpartum depression is to maintain a strong and selfless bond with your baby. The stronger your bond with your baby, the healthier you will be. In the next part, we will take a closer look at the different prenatal tests that are undertaken during pregnancy, and we will start with the Ultrasound in the next chapter.

PART 3

14

ULTRASOUND SCANS DURING PREGNANCY

The first time you visit your Doctor when you are expecting, you will be asked to get an ultrasound scan done. This scan is to check the baby's well-being and monitor the growth inside the womb. Watching their baby during the scanning is one of the happiest experiences for all expectant parents. An ultrasound scan is suggested at around six weeks of pregnancy; these scans are indispensable for the pregnancy. Ideally, two types of scans are done during the first trimester of pregnancy: Early pregnancy scan and Nuchal translucency scan (NT scan). Let us have a detailed look into it.

Early pregnancy scan: It is ideally done between six weeks and eight weeks of pregnancy.

- **Preparation for the scan**: There are two ways to conduct this scan: the transabdominal and transvaginal approaches. Your Doctor or sonologist decides the scan approach.
- **Transabdominal approach**: It is necessary to have a full bladder before the scan to better see the uterus and ovaries. The expectant mother is asked to lie down comfortably, after which a small amount of gel is spread on the belly.

The ultrasound transducer (probe) is run over the stomach to examine the development of the baby. This feels like a massage; however, you may experience a slight discomfort if pressure is applied to the abdomen by the transducer.

- **Transvaginal approach** (TVS): This type of ultrasound scan is done when the pregnancy is too early to be identified through an abdominal scan. TVS is the preferred examination technique if the pregnancy is less than seven weeks. Unlike for the transabdominal approach, you would be asked to empty the bladder before the scan. The Doctor or the nurse will insert a small cylindrical transducer (probe) wrapped with a sterile cover into your vaginal cavity to see the pregnancy. The privacy of the expectant mother is ensured during the scan. Their consent is very important. An expectant mother has the right to either accept or deny the TVS. While undertaking this procedure, you may experience a little pressure on your vagina while moving the probe. However, you will not experience pain unless you are too sensitive or you have vaginismus.

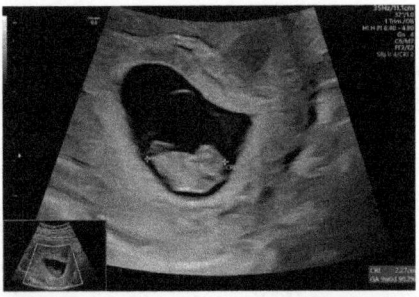

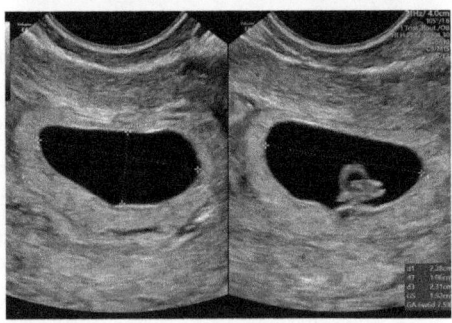

Illustration of early pregnancy scan showing gestation sac, embryo, and yolk sac

DUE DATE

An early pregnancy scan helps in...

- Understanding whether the pregnancy is inside or outside the uterus,
- Estimating the duration of the pregnancy,
- Documenting the heartbeat,
- Confirming the number of pregnancies (single/multiple),
- Evaluating the condition of the uterus and ovaries, and
- Calculating the estimated due date (EDD).

If the early pregnancy scan report is normal, you will be asked to book an appointment for an NT scan unless it warrants any repeat scan before the 12th week.

First Trimester NT Scan

What is an NT ultrasound scan? NT scan, which checks for nuchal translucency, is a screening ultrasound scan conducted to determine the baby's risk of developing chromosomal abnormalities like Down syndrome, Trisomy 13, and Trisomy 18. Also known as a combined screening test, it is done to detect structural abnormalities in the baby.

According to the ISUOG guidelines, the NT scan is strictly performed when the baby is 45–84 mm in length, which corresponds to 11 weeks to 13 weeks six days of pregnancy (before the 14th week). However, the best time to do this scan is from 12–13 weeks. Before the 12th week of gestation, it may be difficult to identify certain structures in the baby since the baby is too small. It is good to choose an experienced Doctor for this scan.

Make sure that your bladder is full before undertaking the procedure. However, as it can take some time, always remember not to fill the bladder completely; it might create discomfort once you start the procedure. No diet restriction is required when you prepare yourself for the scanning procedure.

The scan time depends on the position of the baby. This is a protocol-driven study, and hence, the baby's position is crucial to getting a proper NT scan and nasal bone measurement. If the position is favorable for the scan, the scan is completed in 10–20 minutes.

If the baby's position is not good for the scan, you will be asked to wait so that baby changes its position. The scan is repeated at multiple close intervals of time until an ideal position is obtained to complete the scan. It is advised to schedule your appointment during the first half of the day to have enough time to wait and complete the scan on the same day.

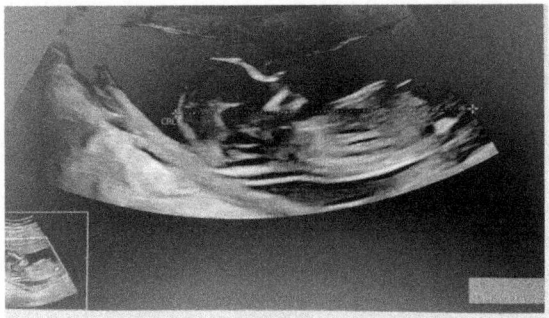

Illustration of first-trimester NT scan

Down syndrome is diagnosed by fluid accumulation, which is found beneath the skin surface and is best appreciated in the neck region. This is called NT. The NT thickness increases in Down syndrome. Any value which is above 3 mm raises the suspicion of having Down syndrome. NT thickness varies with the gestational age of the fetus. However, an increased NT above the 90th centile represents a high risk for chromosomal abnormality. Although abnormal NT thickness is not specific for Down syndrome, further tests are advised to confirm the diagnosis or exclude chromosomal abnormalities.

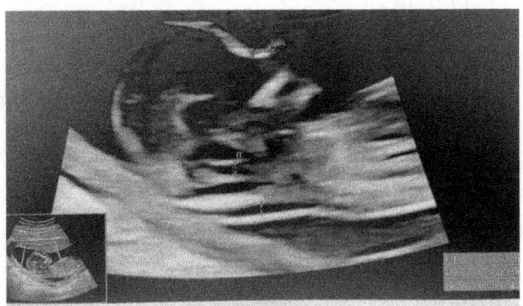

2-D Ultrasound scan showing Nuchal Translucency, Nasal Bone, and Intra-cranial Translucency

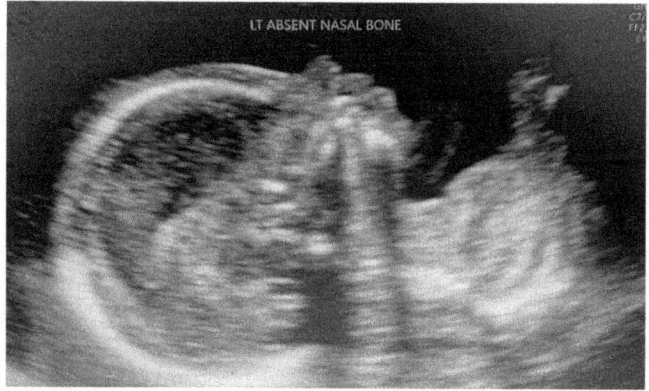

2-D scan with an absent nasal bone

Non-visualization of the nasal bone, absent nasal bone, and unossified nasal bone are different terminologies used in the scan report. This basically means that the nasal bone is not formed. In 65 percent of Down syndrome babies, the nasal bone is not formed. Likewise, five percent of genetically normal babies will not have the nasal bone.

Abnormal nuchal thickness along with absent nasal bone are strong markers for the diagnosis of Down syndrome. It is mandatory to undergo amniocentesis or Non-invasive prenatal diagnostic test (NIPT) to confirm or exclude Down syndrome. Many times, the nasal bone develops at a later stage of pregnancy. Hence, another scan will be done to check the nasal bone at around 16 weeks of pregnancy.

What is the Doppler Study in the First-Trimester Scan?

Doppler assessment of uterine arteries is part of the NT scan. If there is an abnormal placenta formation, the resistance increases in the placental bed. This is seen as increased resistance in one or both uterine arteries as an early diastolic notch. This Doppler study of the uterine artery can predict the chances of developing pregnancy-induced hypertension and fetus growth restriction.

Second-Trimester Ultrasound Scan:

This is also called an anomaly scan or targeted imaging for fetal anomaly scan (TIFFA).

This scan detects the baby's abnormalities, if any, and is important to determine whether pregnancy needs to be continued or terminated. The anomaly scan is recommended at 18 weeks to 20 weeks of pregnancy (at the fifth month).

Most of the fetal structures are formed during this period, and the organs would be seen better. It is good to schedule an appointment for the scan at your convenience. The scan time depends on the position of the baby. The scan time typically lasts for 15–30 minutes. If the baby's position is not favorable for the scan, especially to see the heart, face, spine, and limbs, you will be asked to wait so that the baby changes its position.

Third-Trimester Ultrasound Scan:

The third-trimester ultrasound scan is also known as Growth Scan or Bio-physical Profile Scan (BPS). The growth scan is done during the seventh or eighth month of pregnancy. This scan gives information on the baby's growth (weight) and position, liquor volume, blood flow (Doppler study), and overall well-being (BPS) of the baby inside the uterus. Additionally, a term scan is recommended by some doctors at the ninth month of pregnancy.

There are other optional ultrasound scans like Fetal-echo, Cervical length study, and limited study to check Doppler and liquor volume. These scans are undertaken depending on the mother's and baby's conditions.

It is good to understand the different genetic tests that are often undertaken during pregnancy, like ultrasound scans. So, let us learn about them in the next chapter.

15

PRENATAL GENETIC SCREENING TESTS DURING PREGNANCY

NT scan, anomaly scan, NIPT, double marker, triple marker, and quadruple markers, etc., are the various prenatal screening tests undertaken during pregnancy. We have already discussed the NT scan and anomaly scan in the previous chapter. Now, let us focus on the other types of screening tests. Every parent wishes for a healthy baby. Most of the parents are concerned about their baby's health throughout the pregnancy journey. While most pregnancy outcomes are good, there are some cases with complications. Some babies might be born with disabilities, and these congenital disabilities are primarily due to chromosomal abnormalities during embryo formation.

Before discussing the screening tests, it is good to know about chromosomes and the causes for genetic defects in the baby. Chromosomes are present in every cell of the human body, and they carry genes that determine an individual's physical characteristics. Usually, each cell in our body contains 23 pairs of chromosomes (total 46), and this condition is called *euploidy*. Any variation in the number, structure, or sequence of chromosomes is called *aneuploidy*.

When a sperm meets the egg in the fallopian tube, 23 pairs of chromosomes from each parent fuse to form a 46-chromosome embryo (23 pairs)—any error in mixing these chromosomes during fertilization results in a genetic abnormality in the baby. The genetic abnormality can occur in the form of an extra chromosome (trisomy), less number of chromosomes (deletion), mismatch, mutation, or mixing up (translocation). Any extra pair of chromosomes in the baby is called a **Trisomy**. Remember that all genetic abnormalities need not be expressed as physical or mental defects in the newborn.

At times, when there is a chromosomal complication, spontaneous miscarriage might occur during the early pregnancy period in most cases. Occasionally, a pregnancy might grow even with abnormal genetic composition of the fetus, resulting in a defective or **anomalous** baby. The most common type of chromosomal abnormality is **Trisomy 21** in the general population. This condition is known as **Down syndrome.** Other common problems are **Trisomy 18 (Patau's)** and **Trisomy 13 (Edwards syndrome)**. These are just a few common examples of chromosomal abnormalities. Hundreds and thousands of chromosomal abnormalities exist, which results in congenital disabilities of varying severity.

The screening tests undertaken during pregnancy will help us know the risk of these three common chromosomal conditions in the baby. **Screening tests** help detect health disorders or diseases in people who do not manifest any disease symptoms. A high-risk test result suggests we go for confirmatory tests to clarify the issue. On the other hand, a low-risk test result assures us to continue the pregnancy without worry. However, screening tests are not confirmatory tests for diagnosing a problem, but they warn us to take necessary action to improve the pregnancy outcome.

Screening tests are safe; they are non-invasive and less expensive compared to definitive tests like amniocentesis and karyotyping. Hence, a screening test is done on every pregnant woman to estimate her risk of having a baby with Down syndrome, Trisomy 13, or Trisomy 18. The first cluster of screening tests I wish to discuss with you is the NT scan and Double marker blood test: the scan details have been discussed in the previous chapter. These two tests are done together; hence, they are called the **combined test** for screening.

The triple and quadruple marker blood tests are done between 15 weeks and 20 weeks of pregnancy. An anomaly scan, also called the second-trimester screening scan, is done between 18 weeks and 24 weeks of pregnancy.

First-Trimester Screening - Double Marker Test

As mentioned, an NT scan and Double marker blood test are done simultaneously. The blood test measure two components in the mother's serum:

1. PAPP-A: pregnancy-associated plasma protein
2. hCG: human chorionic gonadotropin

Possible Outcomes of the Combined Tests

These are the possible outcomes:

1. Low-risk NT scan and low-risk double marker test—continue the pregnancy without any worry.
2. Low-risk NT scan and high-risk double marker test—the pregnant woman will be advised to undergo an early anomaly scan at the 16th week.
3. High-risk NT scan and low-risk double marker test—the pregnant woman will be advised to undergo an early anomaly scan at the 16th week. Alternatively, a NIPT test or amniocentesis is advised depending on other risk factors.

Down syndrome expected risk is calculated based on ultrasound findings alone or combined tests (ultrasound & double marker test). The combined test is more reliable for risk assessment. For example, if the result is somewhere between 1:10 and 1:250, it means that the baby lies in a high-risk zone.

Likewise, a risk ratio which is 1:1000 or more means the baby is in a low-risk category. The combined test can detect 85%–87% of pregnancies with Down syndrome. The double marker test will also show the expected risk of the baby having a neural tube defect. A thorough repeat scan needs to be done in the 16th week, if the double marker test shows the presence of risk for neural tube defect.

The Second-Trimester Screening Tests

Ultrasonography

As mentioned in the previous chapter, ultrasonography is a screening test for detecting genetic problems. In this scan, specific subtle soft markers are checked, which are indicative of chromosome abnormality. You might be wondering what these soft markers are?

The soft markers are ultrasound findings in an unborn baby, which are indicative of aneuploidy. The soft markers are also seen in normal karyotype fetuses in a small percentage. Some of the commonly seen soft markers are

1. Choroid plexus cysts in the brain,
2. An echogenic bowel,
3. An aberrant right subclavian artery,
4. Echogenic focus in the baby heart, and so on.

Having the presence of more than one soft marker might suggest a genetic abnormality. However, they are usually found in isolation, and hence there is no need to worry.

Maternal Serum Tests:

Triple marker and quadruple marker blood tests are similar to double marker tests. Suppose you fall under the high-risk category while the test results are obtained. In that case, it suggests that your chance of having a genetically abnormal baby is higher compared to that of the general population.

Non-Invasive Prenatal Testing (NIPT/Cell-Free DNA Testing in Mother)

NIPT is a screening blood test that helps in detecting chromosomal abnormalities in the fetus. NIPT has better sensitivity (95 percent)to detect Down syndrome risk in the baby compared to the Double marker and Quadruple marker blood tests. The test detects the circulating fetus' cell-free DNA component in the mother's blood.

The NIPT test is done any time after 10 weeks of pregnancy. NIPT is a relatively expensive blood test compared to the others. Hence the test is not done on every pregnant woman.

NIPT is suggested under the following circumstances:

- Mother's age is more than 35 years, resulting in a high chance of giving birth to genetically abnormal offspring.
- A previous pregnancy with a defective baby.
- A high-risk category based on NT scan or blood serum markers.
- If the mother is not willing for invasive procedures like amniocentesis or chorionic villus biopsy.

POINTS TO NOTE ABOUT NIPT

- Since NIPT is a screening test, the positive test result should be confirmed with a definitive study like karyotyping.
- NIPT is not suggested in multiple pregnancies (twins or triplets).
- NIPT may rarely give false-positive or false-negative results.

Apart from chromosomal defects (aneuploidy), certain congenital disabilities in the offspring are inherited from the parents or grandparents. The most common disorders are Thalassemia, Cystic fibrosis, Sickle cell anemia, Fragile X syndrome, Duchenne muscular dystrophy, Hemophilia, and Huntington's disease.

One or both parents may carry the defective gene and pass it on to the baby. These genetic disorders run in the family. The affected gene may manifest the disease or only be a carrier without displaying the disease.

It is advised to test the parents for these genetic disorders. The carrier screening blood tests (parental karyotyping) help identify the possibility of the baby being affected by the disease.

Karyotyping

A Karyotyping test is a method to analyze the chromosomes. Any defective chromosome can be identified by karyotyping. It utilizes the amniotic fluid, blood sample, or any other body fluids to check for chromosomal abnormalities. Although karyotyping can be done on any cells from the body, it is usually done on amniotic fluid cells to detect chromosomal abnormalities in the fetus. This is a test that can also be used to detect the chromosomal abnormalities present in adults. The following categories of people are advised to undertake this test.

a. Couples who have experienced repeated miscarriages.
b. People with a family history of genetic diseases.
c. Pregnant women who are at a higher risk of giving birth to babies with genetic disorders. For example, expectant mothers aged 35 and above. Karyotyping can also be used to detect the cause for the intrauterine death of the fetus.

In the next chapter, let us learn about amniocentesis, a procedure often performed for Karyotyping.

16

AMNIOCENTESIS AND CHORIONIC VILLUS SAMPLING (CVS)

I once met a 42-year-old pregnant woman who had approached me during her second pregnancy. She had an elder daughter, who was about 10 years old. The second one was an unplanned pregnancy. The couple learned that the mother's double marker and quadruple marker blood tests indicated a high-risk pregnancy for chromosomal abnormalities. They rushed to my clinic upon receiving their results.

I decided to conduct "amniocentesis" to understand the actual condition of the baby. The day I chose for the procedure was the tenth birthday of their elder daughter. They were planning a grand party; however, the result of the quadruple test troubled them, and they decided to call off the function.

I still remember the expression on the mother's face when she was undertaking the process. She was praying throughout the procedure; once she got out, I took her to our boardroom, where our team had arranged a birthday function for her daughter, which was a surprise for them. Now, you might be wondering why I am sharing this story with you.

It is to remind you that even though you might be going through a challenging phase in your life, the Doctors are always here to support you. Now, coming back to the topic, many women have asked me about the pros and cons of the amniocentesis procedure. So, let us now understand in detail what amniocentesis is and the different steps associated with it.

Amniocentesis:

Amniocentesis is a diagnostic ultrasound-guided procedure where a small quantity of the amniotic fluid is taken from the pregnant uterus. Amniotic fluid contains baby's cells which are shed from their skin surface. These cells carry genetic information about the baby, which in turn helps to diagnose certain genetic and metabolic disorders. The amniotic fluid drawn from the pregnant uterus is sent to the lab for genetic analysis. The cells are separated from the fluid and are cultured and grown for studying their genetic composition. This study is known as Karyotyping, which we have discussed in the previous chapter. Amniocentesis is advised to pregnant women at 15–22 weeks of pregnancy. The indications for the amniocentesis test are discussed in the chapter titled "Prenatal Genetic Tests in Pregnancy". The types of chromosomal tests depend upon the condition suspected in the Ultrasound scans and the clinical history.

The common tests are

- **FISH (Fluorescence in situ hybridization):** This test is particularly done to check for Trisomy 21(Down syndrome), Trisomy 13, Trisomy 18, and Monosomy X.
- **Chromosomal microarray (CMA):** This test detects abnormalities in any 23 pairs of chromosomes.
- **Single-gene testing:** This test is done if the family history or carrier screening shows that the baby might be at risk of a single-gene disorder

The amniocentesis procedure is relatively safe. However, procedure-related miscarriage can happen in 0.1 percent of cases. Other rare and minor complications are mild cramping pain, bleeding, or amniotic fluid leak from the vagina.

I recall meeting Prajitha, who complained about cramping pain after undergoing amniocentesis. After a follow-up scan and thorough physical examination, I confirmed no threat to the pregnancy. The pain subsided after two days of the procedure.

Chorionic Villus Sampling (CVS):

CVS is a transcervical procedure where a small sample of the placenta called a chorionic villus is taken to diagnose chromosomal abnormalities, since the genetic composition of the placenta and the baby is identical. CVS is done under ultrasound guidance and it is an outpatient procedure. The test is done between the tenth and the thirteenth week. CVS is done to detect inborn metabolic errors and inherited genetic disorders in the baby.

Fetal Blood Sampling:

Fetal blood sampling is another way to study the genetic make-up of the baby. This procedure is reserved to know the severity of anemia in the baby in cases of Rh incompatibility. This procedure is usually done after 18 weeks of pregnancy. In the next part, let us look at the pregnancy calendar and learn what to expect at each phase when you are pregnant.

PART 4

17

PREGNANCY CALENDAR: FIRST MONTH

The first four weeks of pregnancy constitute the first month of pregnancy. The baby is not yet formed in this phase, and your body is preparing for the pregnancy. The missed menstrual cycle is the first predictive sign of pregnancy. Some women experience PMS-like early pregnancy symptoms, which include mood swings, bloating, and abdomen cramps. This is the phase where the uterus gets prepared to accept the fertilized egg.

Usually, the first day of your last menstrual date is considered the starting day of your 40-week pregnancy period. You have ovulated in the 3rd week of the first month, symbolized by the hike in the basal body temperature. Soon after the ovulation, the egg released from your fallopian tube gets fertilized by your partner's sperm. This fertilized egg is called the zygote.

Once the fertilization is completed, and the zygote is formed, several mutations happen within the zygote, and it starts to divide into clusters of multiple cells. These cells move into the uterus for implantation. Implantation is accompanied by light scanty bleeding or spotting in vagina in 25 percent of the cases. This bleeding is known as implantation bleeding. Do not panic about this bleeding, as it will settle down.

The fertilized egg secretes hCG, a pregnancy hormone responsible for positive pregnancy tests in urine and blood tests. Soon after the implantation, your baby is now in embryo form. An embryo is a microscopic structure within the uterus. A missed period gives you the sign that you are pregnant, and hence, the first month is often unidentified during a pregnancy journey. Some women do complain about nausea, food aversions, etc., but, most often these symptoms are ignored. Hence, even though the pregnancy journey starts from the first month onwards, the real excitement and discomfort associated with this phase begin only in the second month.

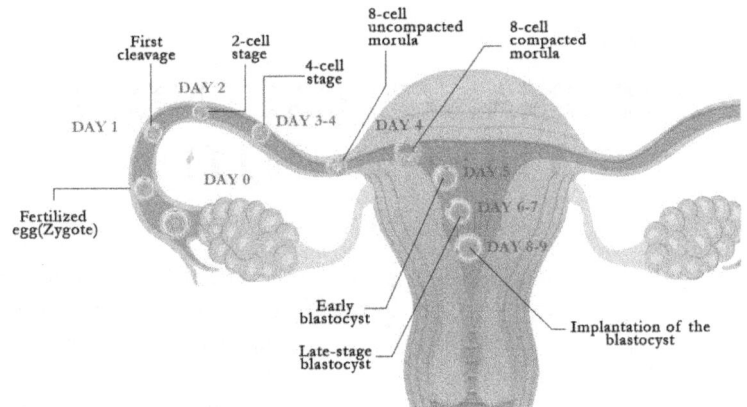

Pictorial diagram depicting Fertilization and Implantation

Some major tips to be undertaken during this period of pregnancy include the following.

- Avoid alcohol and quit smoking.
- Start vitamin supplements for increasing the chances of fertility.
- Consuming 400 µg of folic acid daily during this month reduces the risk of neural tube defects in unborn babies.

We will discuss the different phases of pregnancy in the following chapters.

18

PREGNANCY CALENDAR: SECOND MONTH

Fatigue, nausea, frequent urination, dizziness, food aversion, and food cravings are some of the symptoms experienced during your second month of pregnancy, which spans from the 5th week to the 8th week. It is during this phase that the good news is revealed.

Sonal, a patient of mine, had an irregular menstrual cycle. She used to experience extensive bleeding, and the medicines prescribed by her Doctors did not help to reduce the bleeding. She was finally given a shot of depot medroxyprogesterone acetate, a hormonal injection to stop menstrual bleeding.

This treatment worked, and she was later sent to me for an ultrasound scan to diagnose the underlying issue.

Apart from the polycystic ovaries, Sonal had nothing to worry about. Patients like Sonal find it difficult to identify pregnancy in the first month. However, one final day, Sonal came to me bearing the good news. She was about two and a half months pregnant when the tests were confirmed. The second month is when pregnancies are diagnosed. You confirm your pregnancy with home-based tests (UPT) or by a blood test. It would be best to visit the Doctor once your home test comes out positive. The gestation sac appears as a dark spot within the uterus.

The embryo ranges in size from a lemon seed to a full-size lemon between week five and week nine. You will be able to hear your baby's heartbeat between week six and week seven. You need not be surprised if your scanning Doctor tells you the heartbeat has not appeared; this usually happens if you get the scan before six weeks. You may have to come back for the scan after two weeks to confirm the pregnancy's viability. It is suggested to get your first pregnancy scan done between six weeks and seven weeks.

The baby develops all facial features (mouth, tongue, and nose) in the second month. The eyelids, though formed during this phase, will be closed throughout much of the pregnancy period. Along with fingers, the toenails also develop during this phase. The baby would have started moving inside the womb, although the expectant mother might not feel it. The baby will also develop different organs, skeletal structures, and limbs once the second month is completed.

Colleen de Bellefonds, a contributing editor/writer at What to Expect, says pregnancy is like "climbing a mountain without training while carrying a backpack that weighs a little more every day." This is true. The first sign of pregnancy is **fatigue**. It takes a lot of energy to assist the baby's growth inside the womb. The mother's body requires a lot of energy and nutrients to form the placenta, a life support system for the baby inside your womb. Thus, fatigue sets in soon after you conceive. Working women often miss this sign.

Smell sensitivity is the next sign you might experience during the early phase of pregnancy. I recall my neighbor, Arathy, asking my wife whether she had cooked paneer for dinner. She was unaware that she was pregnant, and one night my wife got a call from her. Arathy called and asked my wife if we had cooked paneer for dinner. My wife was shocked as Arathy stayed four blocks from our home. Our neighbors did not inquire about paneer, and my wife had commented that they might have had nasal congestion. However, I, on the other hand, remarked that Arathy could be pregnant. Two weeks after this incident, my wife asked me if I had learned astrology, as my prediction was accurate. Arathy was four weeks pregnant at that time.

If you feel nauseous, do not blame the food you consume or the cook who prepared the food. The credit, instead, should go to your partner, who has given you the best present in the world. **Morning sickness** is an irritating sign that comes with the onset of pregnancy. Many myths revolve around this single sign of pregnancy.

I had a patient named Kavitha, who was very thrilled to welcome her son. When I asked how she was so sure it was a son, she replied that her morning sickness in the first three months was a sign that she was carrying a son. I was not ready to argue with her as she was the last patient that day. She continued expounding on the relationship between morning sickness and the gender of the child. Later she told me that all the women in her family, who had experienced morning sickness, gave birth to sons. This is definitely a coincidence. I have seen women with severe morning sickness giving birth to baby girls. Be careful about such myths and make sure not to get captivated by such unscientific claims.

Food aversions become a problem for pregnant women. My friend, a Doctor herself, talked about her struggles when she was expecting during an inspiring online session on pregnancy. She always loved fried fish. With the coming of pregnancy, the smell of fried fish irritated her. She used to have nightmares about strangers forcing her to eat fried fish. That session was an eye-opener. Many people miss out on these evident signs of pregnancy.

Another pregnancy symptom we always associate with the hike in hormone levels is ***mood swings***. It is a challenging task to predict when and how the mood of a pregnant woman will change. I have seen many husbands complaining about their wives' mood swings. If you ask me, the husbands have to understand the pain and sufferings women go through preparing their bodies to shelter a baby. The fathers-to-be must understand the hardships endured by women. I had met Sandeep, who often complained about his wife's sudden mood swings. He stated an incident where the couple watched the movie 'Kal Ho Naa Ho,' and his wife cried throughout the second half of the show. He asked me if this was a common phenomenon. As I could not advise him at that point, I asked him to inform the Gynecologist. If you feel depressed or irritated, it is good to inform your Gynecologist.

Tender or swollen breasts are another sign of pregnancy. You might feel the sudden need to change your bra to a larger size. Sometimes, you might feel suffocated wearing a favorite dress, which was fine the previous week. Breast changes are a sure sign of pregnancy. Along with breast tenderness, you might also see your areolas in a darker shade. It is crucial to have a closer look at yourself if you are planning a pregnancy. Most of the changes that come with pregnancy can only be identified by you.

You might feel irritated to visit the washroom frequently during your working hours. However, the need to urinate more regularly will become a pattern until delivery. This ***urgency to urinate*** will start as early as the second or third week of the pregnancy. The pregnancy hormone Beta-hCG is the real cause for this sudden change. Beta-hCG tends to increase blood flow to the kidneys to remove all the toxic elements entering the body.

Along with this, the enlarging uterus exerts pressure on the bladder, resulting in less storage space for urine. Both these components together cause an urgency to urinate. Be on guard, as frequent urination can also be a sign of urinary tract infection and diabetes.

Bloating and high body basal temperature are some of the other symptoms you can expect during the first months of pregnancy. Hence, all these signs and symptoms are referred to as early pregnancy symptoms; most of them vanish when you enter the second trimester, which spans from the fourth month to the sixth month.

I recommend pre-pregnancy counseling to all couples planning a baby. Usually, in such counseling sessions, the counselor informs the couple about the signs and symptoms of pregnancy, and the various changes that can happen to a woman's body during pregnancy. The Doctors often advise the husbands to ensure that their wives have a comfortable and tension-free pregnancy. Possessing sound knowledge about what to expect when you are expecting will prepare a couple to face all the hardships and issues of pregnancy. After all, the love and care for each other is the sole strength that will drive them through this phase.

Once you confirm your pregnancy, you should make it a point to schedule an appointment with your Doctor at the earliest. I remember meeting a couple who expressed their worries over their unborn child. This was her second pregnancy, as she had suffered a miscarriage earlier. The couple blamed themselves for that devastating incident as they had postponed the Doctor's appointment due to their tight and busy work schedule. Whenever they met a pregnant woman, they always made it a point to advice on the importance of frequent visits to the Doctor during pregnancy. You might feel that medical check-ups are unnecessary during pregnancy as you need more rest than to and fro visits to the clinic.

Nevertheless, these check-ups will enable you to maintain the correct weight, blood sugar levels, and blood pressure levels. If these counts are not within the normal range, you might have many complications during pregnancy, including gestational diabetes, pre-eclampsia, and overweight. It is good to have an understanding of these medical conditions. Along with the signs and symptoms of pregnancy mentioned earlier, you will likely develop some other symptoms also this month. The sudden increase in hormone levels can lead to increased *vaginal discharge*. The renowned pregnancy glow occurs during this phase as well.

However, some women can develop **severe acne** problems during this time. One of my friends, Dr. Rajam, informed me about a patient who complained about an increased amount of whitish vaginal discharge. This patient was scared, and Dr. Rajam tried to calm her down by informing her that it was normal during pregnancy. As the patient was not ready to believe this, she was sent to me for a scan. She was sobbing when she entered the scanning room and asked me if I had dealt with women who had suffered a miscarriage. I was shocked to hear this from her and comforted her by revealing that her baby was healthy. She then asked about her discharge; however, I was not able to clarify and dispel all her doubts.

Some days after this incident, I met Dr. Rajam, who told me the patient had initially researched the pregnancy symptoms, but was now convinced that nothing was wrong. Maybe after all that research, she had become an expert herself. I always advise pregnant women to research the signs, symptoms, and discomforts of pregnancy to understand what is happening in their bodies. The better understanding you have, the happier you will be. A **stuffy nose** is another pregnancy symptom that you might encounter during the second month.

In such cases, do not blame the immediate change in surroundings. This condition is caused by the sudden increase of estrogen and progesterone in the body. You may also suddenly find out that you are **no longer shedding hair**. You might wonder how you were successful in eliminating hair fall. Do not try to congratulate your hairdresser or your hair specialist. The absence of hair fall is solely due to the incredible work of pregnancy hormones present in your body. Sadly, after three months of delivery, you will experience hair fall.

My cousin Radhika had long and thick hair when she was planning for pregnancy. However, she decided to cut her hair during her pregnancy as she thought it might hinder her daily activities. By the time she stopped feeding her baby, her hair had grown back. However, she soon started experiencing unexpected hair fall. The second month marks the beginning of your frequent visits to your Gynecologist. This is also a time for your Doctor to know more about you as they might ask you questions about your medical history, your family's medical history, your job, and so on. The Doctor does so to spot the potential risks you might encounter during your pregnancy.

During this month, you will also be asked to run urine and blood tests to confirm the pregnancy and identify the possible threats to your pregnancy. You will also be asked to undergo an ultrasound scan to confirm the location of pregnancy and check for uterine and ovarian cysts.

The Doctors make it a point to check the abdomen. As a usual procedure, the Doctors will check your blood pressure, height, and weight. During pregnancy, your blood pressure should not exceed 130/90 mmHg. A higher value might lead to pregnancy issues such as pre-eclampsia, decreased blood flow to the placenta, intrauterine baby growth restriction, etc. It is assumed that pregnant women are likely to gain 1 kg per month during their first trimester.

However, there are cases where pregnancy might lead to weight reduction. In case you gain an excessive amount of weight during the first trimester, you must definitely inform your Gynecologist about this, as excessive weight gain in pregnancy can lead to pre-eclampsia, liver and kidney problems, placental abruption, and other complications.

I would also like to enlighten you about some of the blood tests and urine tests conducted during this phase. Urine tests are mainly done to check the presence of protein and sugar in the urine. It also helps in identifying the presence of pus cells, which confirms urinary tract infection. If the sample contains traces of protein, it suggests that you might have kidney problems. The presence of sugar, on the other hand, is a sign of diabetes.

Many pregnant women are diagnosed with urinary tract infections and vaginal infections, mostly diagnosed with urine routine tests. Some of the essential laboratory tests to be taken during the second month include Complete Blood Count (CBC),

Blood grouping and Rh typing, tests for infectious diseases such as HIV, Hepatitis A, Hepatitis B, or Hepatitis C, VDRL, HbA1c, and Thyroid Function Test. These tests are called the Antenatal Care (ANC) profile. Blood grouping and Rh typing are essential if blood transfusion is needed in case of blood loss during delivery or surgery. One of my friends, named Sudha, came to see me for her early pregnancy scan.

She was thrilled to talk about the different changes happening to her body, and I lectured her about the need to do blood tests. After the lecture, I asked her about the blood test results, and she told me that everything was fine and normal. I enquired about her rubella result, and she replied that it was negative and hence she was feeling relaxed.

I could not help her at that time as she was already seven weeks pregnant. Then I realized that many women are unaware of rubella vaccination, and also of the fact that if they got vaccinated for rubella, the blood test result would be positive for the same. Indeed, a positive rubella test shows that you are immune to the disease. It is always good to check for rubella during the planning time itself.

I hope this information will be helpful for you in your journey. I would also like to provide some insights into the different procedures that are often undertaken during pregnancy. In fact, when you approach the Doctor after getting a positive test result in your pregnancy test, your Doctor will inform you about these tests, which need to be undertaken for a safe pregnancy.

The table provided below will give you an idea of the different tests undertaken during all three trimesters of pregnancy.

Sl. No.	Corresponding Weeks in Pregnancy	Tests to be Undertaken
1.	Before 12th week	ANC Profile Early Pregnancy Scan (EP scan)
2.	12–13 weeks	NT scan (Nuchal Translucency scan) For checking Down Syndrome Double marker test Blood tests for assessing

		Iron and Calcium Blood test to assess the range of TSH
3.	16 weeks	Glucose Challenge Test (if you are diabetic) Clinical Check-up
4.	20 weeks	Anomaly Scan The first dose of Tetanus will be administered
5.	24 weeks	Clinical Check-up Complete Blood Count Urine Routine and Microscopy
6.	26 weeks	Clinical Check-up Oral Glucose Tolerance Test
7.	28–30 weeks	Growth scan Boostrix injection The second dose of Tetanus
8.	34–37 weeks	Blood tests
9.	37th week	End term scan
10.	40th week	Full term

Let us also analyze some strategies you could take up for the Maternal-Child Health (MCH) care. It is interesting to note that these strategies are often termed the "12 to 1" strategies of MCH care.

	Strategy
12	Make sure to do the antenatal registration before you complete **12** weeks.
11	Your haemoglobin level should be **11** gm% or above throughout your pregnancy.
10	Ensure that your weight gain from conception till delivery is **10** kg
09	Try to obtain good care and practise self-care throughout the **9** months of pregnancy.

DUE DATE

08	You should have at least **8** visits during your antenatal period.
07	Your Doctor would advise a blood transfusion if your Hb level is **7** gm% or below.
06	There are **6** major tests that needs to be taken during pregnancy- Hb, Hep. B, VDRL, HIV, Albumin, Thyroid. You should undertake at least **6** weeks of minimum postnatal care. Also, try to exclusively breastfeed your baby for the first **6** months.
05	The anomaly scan is usually conducted during the **5**th month.
04	Ensure to plot the cervical Partogram from **4** cm of dilation.
03	If you are diabetic before pregnancy or have a strong family history of Diabetes, ensure to take Glucose Challenge Test, at least **3** times during your pregnancy.
02	There are **2** doses of tetanus vaccination that you need to take during pregnancy.
01	Before taking any decision regarding your pregnancy, ensure to get at least 1 expert opinion and **1** complete blood count.

Having equipped ourselves with ample knowledge, let us now move on to the next month, the third month of pregnancy, which marks the end of the first trimester.

19

PREGNANCY CALENDAR: THIRD MONTH

The third month of pregnancy, which corresponds to the 9th to 13th weeks of pregnancy, marks the end of the first trimester. If you were expecting a little comfort in your third month, you better gear up; the third month will be a rollercoaster ride.

While the morning sickness might ease out for a few, many expectant mothers have an increased appetite during the third month. The growing placenta secretes a higher amount of hCG hormone, creating more discomfort during this month. Some of the major discomforts experienced during this period include excess fatigue, bloating and burping sensation, and nausea.

When you reach the third month, there are chances of experiencing an increase in nausea due to the effect of progesterone on your stomach and gut muscles. This might lead to severe food aversions and weakness. Tackling nausea is very different, and during pregnancy, many women consider this a real obstacle to peace. Avoiding eating will only lead to severe pregnancy issues, so include plenty of dried fruits, nuts, and energy-boosting snacks in your meal; this will help you overcome nausea and fatigue. Eight years ago, I met a pregnant woman in the casualty department who had tried to commit suicide.

As senior Doctors were not available, I was asked to attend to her and calm her down. When I entered her cubicle, I saw a woman with a big dressing on her wrist; she had tried to cut her veins. Her vitals were normal, and hence I started a pleasant conversation with her. I enquired about her family members, and she started crying. I called the other medical attendees to calm her down, and I left her cubicle.

One of the nurses approached me and told me that her mother-in-law was teasing her as her womb had not grown bigger over the previous month. I was shocked and asked myself if she was carrying a giant to have a visible abdomen in the third month. I went out to meet the family, and her mother-in-law was also present, to my surprise. Her husband inquired about her condition and narrated the incident that led to this mishap. I told him to ask his mother whether her abdomen was prominent during the third month. He had no answers and went back and sat on a chair in the waiting area.

If you have a misconception that the baby bump will be visible from the first trimester itself, then you are wrong. Many women will start showing their baby bump only after the 12th week. If you have a lean stature, the baby bump will be more prominent. Some women start showing it earlier. In fact, the visibility of the baby bump depends on the type of body the mother has.

The third month also includes some major ultrasound scanning procedures like First-trimester screening and nuchal translucency (NT) scan. NT scan is sometimes referred to as the NT/NB (nasal bone) scan and helps to rule out chromosomal abnormalities like Down Syndrome or any structural abnormality in the growing baby. The NT scan is performed to check for the presence of the nasal bone and the thickness of the nuchal fold in the baby. If the nasal bone is absent or there is an overly thickened nuchal fold, it indicates Down Syndrome. An NT/NB scan is done along with a blood test named double marker test. Like the scans, a double marker blood test is also done to check for chromosomal issues.

The results of all these are put together to confirm the odds of chromosomal problems in the baby. Hence, every pregnant woman should be aware of these tests and should compulsorily undertake them. Sometimes an NT/NB scan takes more time if the baby's position is not favorable for the scan. So, be prepared to schedule an appointment and take a day off for this scan. I have done the NT/NB scan at multiple sittings for a woman due to the baby's unfavorable position. In such cases, I inform the patients to come the next day to complete the scan. NT scan is a protocol-based study that demands the appropriate position of the baby.

I hope you are now aware of the various changes your body will go through during the first three months of pregnancy. Now, let us move on to the next chapter, the fourth month of pregnancy.

20

PREGNANCY CALENDAR: FOURTH MONTH

The fourth month of the pregnancy spans from the 14th week to the 17th week. Drastic changes happen to the baby inside the uterus during this time, and the baby bump is evident. However, there is no need to panic if the pregnancy bump is not visible by this time.

Many pregnant women *expect* to experience the baby's movements once they reach the fourth month. In reality, they will experience it when they enter or complete the fifth month of pregnancy. I recall a patient named Mileena, who came to see me when she was four months pregnant. She had come for a repeat ultrasound scan as she was doubtful whether her baby was okay or not. When she went for her monthly check-up, her Doctor informed her that the baby was doing fine. Even though her Obstetrician tried to convey that it is normal not to experience the movements in the fourth month, she was not convinced. Hence, to avoid a panicky situation, her Doctor suggested a repeat ultrasound scan, and she was sent to me for the procedure. During the scan, she started shooting questions at me like a CBI officer. But when she heard the baby's heartbeat and saw the baby's movements, she calmed down. The notion that pregnant women must experience the baby's movements in the fourth month is nothing but a total myth.

For some pregnant women, ultrasound scans are repeated in the fourth month if the baby's nasal bone is not visible in the first scan. A lack of nasal bone in the fourth month suggests a high chance of the baby having chromosomal abnormalities. The ultrasonography result is then analyzed along with a triple marker test or quadruple marker blood test to assess the risk of carrying a baby with Down syndrome. The ultrasound scan and blood tests help identify the risk of the baby having Down, Edwards', or Patau syndrome, and they also detect open neural tube defects. Amniocentesis is another test that is used to confirm chromosomal abnormalities. I have seen many women undertake this test to rule out all the chromosomal issues that may be present. I have conducted several amniocentesis tests regularly in our lab.

The fourth month is a pleasant month for many pregnant women as most of the discomforts experienced during the first trimester lessen during this phase. Nausea, vomiting, and dizziness will make way for other discomforts such as heartburn and constipation. It is essential to understand that with the progress of the pregnancy, the discomforts change.

I remember meeting Anuradha, who was four months pregnant. She doubted whether her pregnancy had stopped as her first trimester symptoms were absent when she entered the fourth month. Some of the significant discomforts experienced during the fourth month are indigestion, which leads to acid reflux and heartburn. Women will also experience body pain, specifically backache. They may also experience stretch marks on the abdomen and breast, followed by spider web-like varicose veins. Other discomforts may include a stuffy nose, teeth issues, especially bleeding gums, constipation, indigestion, and round ligament pain that affects the muscles of the pelvis.

At four months, your baby will be the size of a butter fruit. The fetus develops its reproductive organs, hair follicles, and muscle strength during this period. Foremost among them, the fetus's eyes and ears develop this month, enabling it to hear you from inside the womb.

It is good to engage in conversation with your baby as this will help the baby distinguish your voice from others. Singing good songs will also elevate the mood of the baby. In the coming months, sometimes, you will be able to feel the baby's movements when you sing or speak to it.

Some of the major threats to pregnancy during the fourth month include abortion, which can occur due to an incompetent cervix, autoimmune diseases such as lupus or scleroderma, chromosomal abnormalities of the fetus, and placental abruption.

I had a patient who was diagnosed with an incompetent cervix in the fourth month. She was rushed to the hospital as she experienced spotting. She knew that spotting and mild bleeding were uncommon in pregnancy. When I did the scan, I found that the cervix was 2 cm long, when it should have been 3 cm in length or more. I informed the Doctor about the case, and she was immediately taken to the labor room for a minor surgical procedure called cervical cerclage to avoid preterm labor. They put a suture in the opening of the cervix and thus saved the pregnancy.

After a scan, I always advise my patients to check for any symptoms that could threaten their pregnancy, like vaginal bleeding, stomach pain, and severe tightness of the lower tummy. You will be feeling more relaxed as the absence of nausea helps you in improving your appetite. However, you would be distressed on realizing that your favorite clothes do not fit you properly anymore. This, in fact, has a brighter side, as this calls for a new shopping trip with your spouse. Round ligament pain, the newly emerged discomfort of this month, will start to create more troubling experiences for you.

Another major threat you should be aware of during this phase is your body's immune response. Immune response during pregnancy would be very low, and hence it is very important to maintain personal hygiene to be in good health. Therefore, it is very important to practice the following to be healthy during this phase.

1. Wash hands frequently
2. Carry hand sanitizers always
3. Avoid sharing drinks and food
4. Avoid sick people

In the next chapter, we will learn about the changes that come about in the fifth month of pregnancy.

21

PREGNANCY CALENDAR: FIFTH MONTH

The fifth month of pregnancy spans from the 18th week to the 22nd week. Indeed, it is a calm phase for many women, as most of the discomforts they experienced in the previous months settle down, giving rise to newer but fewer discomforts. I recall meeting Nandana, a five-month pregnant woman, who came to my clinic before meeting her Obstetrician. She was sobbing while sitting in the waiting area. One of my staff members, who saw this, informed me, and I called Nandana's husband to know about her issues. I learned that Nandana had conceived after years of treatment. She was scared as she experienced sudden pains in her right pelvic region, similar to the premenstrual cramps. She rushed to the clinic to take an ultrasound scan to ensure her baby was alright, and then planned to meet her Doctor.

As both the husband and wife seemed beset with panic, I decided to conduct an ultrasound scan on priority, even without the Doctor's prescription. Her scan results were perfectly ok, and I showed Nandana her baby on the ultrasound screen. I could see tears rolling down her cheeks; she was relieved. After the scanning procedure, I asked them whether they were aware of the discomforts during pregnancy.

Nandana did not have any discomforts in the first four months, and the sudden pain was a shock for them. I tried to educate them about round ligament pain, a common phenomenon during the fifth month. Many women who come for their scans often complain about pelvic pain and request that I double-check whether everything is ok. Even though an ultrasound scan will not reveal any abnormality associated with round ligament pain, it is advisable to take a scan to rule out other causes of pain, like gall bladder stones, kidney stones, appendicitis, and ovary cysts.

You might be wondering why pregnant women panic when they experience pain during pregnancy. Round ligament pain is very different from other pains and aches you feel during pregnancy. It is a sharp, achy pain that changes with the change in position and is often felt in the lower abdomen or groin area. Some women have the pain only on one side, but others might experience on both the sides.

A group of thick ligaments supports the uterus, and one among them is the round ligament, which connects the sides of the uterus to the groin area. As the baby grows, the round ligament stretches to give extra support to the growing womb. The pregnant woman's sudden movements might result in the ligaments' sudden tightening, which ultimately causes severe pain in the pelvic and groin area. It will only last for a few minutes for some, whereas it might go on for hours for others.

However, all the pain that you experience in the lower abdomen may not be round ligament pain. Sometimes indigestion might create pain in the entire abdomen. If the lower abdomen pain is followed by mild bleeding, spotting, dizziness, nausea, or vomiting, you should rush to your Obstetrician immediately.

Another discomfort that will severely affect you during this phase is fatigue. The baby inside your body is growing at a high-speed mode to accomplish the milestones, and for this purpose, it is using the energy you have.

I heard it from my wife, who was pregnant at the time of writing this book. She told me that she felt as if someone was drinking her life energy. This kind of severe fatigue might be irritating to you. One of my patients, named Rudra, who came for her anomaly scan, commented that she had experienced several episodes of dozing off at her workplace. She reasoned that she was not fired yet because her boss was a woman and knew her situation.

Dozing off, absent-mindedness, inability to concentrate, and excessive feelings of thirst and hunger are all the by-products of fatigue. My professor at the medical college, Dr. Sally Mary, once stated that pregnancy comes with a large package of small discomforts. As the pregnancy progresses, these small discomforts invite their friends and acquaintances for company. This comment turned the whole class into a laughing club. When I see the different cases I encounter, I realize that what she said has been true all this time, "Pregnancy is a large package of small discomforts."

The fifth month is when you undertake the anomaly scan, otherwise termed the mid-pregnancy scan or TIFFA scan. It gives a correct understanding of the physical structures of your baby. This scan also gives you information on the position of the placenta, baby weight and growth, and amniotic fluid levels. The priority of the scan is to detect structural abnormalities in the baby. An anomaly scan usually takes a little longer time than other routine ultrasound scans; hence, block your appointment for the scan so that your Doctor spends a good amount of time studying your baby.

I had a patient named Renuka, who used to come for her pregnancy scans. I specifically remember an incident when we were undertaking her anomaly scan. The baby was not in a good position for the scan, and it took more than half an hour to do the scan. Once the procedure was over, I decided to call her husband, Raghu, to show him the baby. Raghu was so happy to see the baby and thanked me for giving him the opportunity. As soon as he spoke, I noticed a change in the baby. The baby was lying on one side during the procedure, and when Raghu spoke, it raised its hand and turned to the other side.

I told Raghu to say some more words, and as the conversation progressed, we saw the baby moving. All the three of us were thrilled to see the baby's bonding with the father. When Renuka came for her next scan, she informed that Raghu had started being closer to the baby after that incident. I always wonder why hospitals and some scanning centers never allow husbands to enter the scanning room. When they see the baby inside the womb, they will get more attached to it, which is good for the pregnant woman and the baby. An *anomaly scan* is ideally done between the 19th and 20th weeks. All the structural abnormalities cannot be detected in an anomaly scan; there are limitations to the study, and subtle structural problems can be missed easily.

Some defects appear during the latter part of the pregnancy; baby positions may limit the view of the organ for a complete evaluation. Since it is a critical scan during pregnancy, it is advised to choose a good scanning Doctor.

Your Obstetrician will look at the anomaly scan results and other blood counts during your fifth-month check-up. One of my friends checked her thyroid every month as she had suffered a previous miscarriage due to severe hypothyroidism. She was on medicines for her thyroid deficiency; however, she forgot to mention this medical condition to her Obstetrician when she went for consultations. Later, when she suffered a miscarriage, the Doctor suggested checking for thyroid issues. Then she informed the Doctor that she had been taking medication for her thyroid problem. Pregnancy is a period when all your medical issues flare-up. Hence it is essential to mention your medical conditions and any familial medical issues to the Doctor at the very beginning.

A year ago, I attended an online webinar on Gestational Diabetes Mellitus (GDM) conducted by FOGSI (The Federation of Obstetric and Gynaecological Societies of India). One of the speakers, Dr. Mridul Shenoy, mentioned that pregnant women with a strong diabetic tendency or a strong familial history of Diabetes would develop GDM in the fourth or fifth month of pregnancy, even before testing with the Glucose Tolerance Test (GTT). He mentioned several women he had met in the past who had similar situations. This statement reminded me of a patient named Rubiya, who had a large baby bump. During the scanning session, I noticed excess fluid in the womb, and hence I requested her to check the blood glucose level as she was unaware of a diabetic condition till that time.

The glucose test showed a high blood sugar level, and hence her Obstetrician advised her to undertake a GTT. If GDM is not detected early, it might lead to preterm labor and complications. GDM will be discussed in detail in a separate chapter for your understanding.

Many Obstetricians advise their patients to undertake a Quadruple marker test or a Quad Screen test. This test helps detect chromosomal abnormalities in babies. In India, termination of pregnancy is allowed only till the 24th week. Once the mother crosses the 24th week, abortion is not permitted. That is why it is good to confirm a healthy pregnancy before the 24th week.

This is why any structural and chromosomal defects should be detected before 24 weeks of pregnancy. The fifth month is when many pregnant women start pregnancy exercises to strengthen the pelvic area for delivery. Women, who have severe medical conditions like cervical incompetence or placenta previa, are not permitted to do exercises like squats, sit-ups, etc., as it might create complications.

Travelling is also allowed from the fourth month to the sixth month, as it is a much safer period during pregnancy. In the fifth month, a white cheese-like substance called vernix caseosa will cover your baby's body, protecting the skin from prolonged exposure to the amniotic fluid. However, just before birth, this substance sheds out from the body of the baby. During this phase, you will probably experience active and strong kicking, a real feeling of having another life within the body. Yet, these kicks will not be periodic at this time. Hence, if you do not feel the kicks throughout the day, do not panic. Obstetricians suggest that you should check the movements thrice a day, soon after the main meals.

The fifth month has always been an exciting phase during the pregnancy journey, especially as it is when the mother will start experiencing the kick of the baby. In the next chapter, let us discuss the changes when you move from the fifth to the sixth month.

22

PREGNANCY CALENDAR: SIXTH MONTH

The sixth month marks the end of the second trimester, and it extends from the 23rd week to the 27th week. One of my patients, Ramani, visited me at my residence one day and acknowledged the services I had provided as a Doctor during her pregnancy. As we were speaking, I informed her that I was planning on writing a book on pregnancy based on my interactions with different pregnant women.

She was delighted and gave me insights into her own pregnancy. Ramani told me that her second trimester was the best phase of her pregnancy. In the first trimester, she was restricted from traveling; however, due to the Covid pandemic, her company insisted on a "work from home" option. Ramani is an outgoing person, and she hated staying home during this beautiful phase of her life. She wanted to go out and share every moment of it with her friends and colleagues. However, after she crossed the first trimester, her Doctor permitted her to travel, and she wished to resume her offline work, which was not possible during the pandemic. Hence, her husband took her for their long-awaited Ooty trip during her second trimester. So, in short, the second trimester was one of the happiest phases of pregnancy for Ramani.

Before she concluded, she told me something. "Every woman should make their dreams come true during this phase. Once they cross the sixth month, they will experience a lot more restrictions than what they had in their first trimester. The sixth month is a gateway for a constricted life."

I could not wholeheartedly agree with Ramani's comments and views; however, it is true that once you complete the sixth month, you might experience a lot more restrictions as your baby needs more energy, in turn, rendering you exhausted. So, when you are in the sixth month of your pregnancy, enjoy it to the fullest by living your dreams. It is essential to make sure that your dreams are not too adventurous as that might create other issues with your pregnancy.

One of the major issues that you will face in your sixth month of pregnancy will be your inability to wear your once 'most praised and hailed' party dresses. Your baby bump will be evident, and you may not be able to perform several physical activities. I had a patient named Saraswathy, who was very happy with her baby bump, even though she could not wear her favorite dresses. She used to travel by bus, and once she reached the sixth month, some visible changes were experienced in the behavior of her co-travelers. Once she hit the sixth month and had a visible baby bump, the passengers in the bus gave up their seats and made sure she had a comfortable ride. Thus, for Saraswathy, the visibility of her baby bump was a blessing in disguise. Others may feel very awkward about the state of their bodies during pregnancy. I have seen many such cases.

I once had a celebrity patient who was a model. She visited me for her scans often. Having a baby made her very happy, and she felt blessed. However, she could not cope with the changes happening to her body, which included enlarged breasts and the stretch marks on her growing belly and breasts. She was concerned if the stretch marks would remain even after her delivery. I gave her a detailed class on how things would change over time. Although she was not comfortable with her body initially, the thought of having a baby in her arms in a few months made her forget everything. She told me, "Doctor, I sometimes feel sad looking at the state of my body. Nevertheless, whenever I feel the baby's kick, I realize that motherhood is more precious than anything else in the world." Well, if you are someone who is also concerned with your body image during pregnancy, relax, you are not alone.

The sixth month is when you choose a birthing method: delivering the baby at a hospital or a birthing center. There are a few essential things you need to check before choosing a hospital. Always look for centers that have proper neonatal care facilities.

If there is a pregnancy issue from the beginning, it is always good to select a hospital that has an excellent neonatal intensive care unit (ICU). Try to choose a hospital which is close to your residence. It will be tough to travel longer distances when the pain starts. So, a nearby hospital will be better than one farther away. It is always good to opt for a hospital that provides complete maternity services, including antenatal classes, counseling, screening, etc. Your selection screening should also check for the availability of experienced medical practitioners including Anesthesiologists, Obstetricians, and Multidisciplinary Doctors, the hospital's hygiene, etc. So, when you select the birthing center, kindly keep all these factors in mind. Many women prefer having a normal vaginal delivery; however, there are cases where this is not possible.

The sixth month is also a time to undergo the Glucose tolerance test (GTT). Some women who have high blood sugar levels manifest symptoms in the form of painful boils, accumulation of pus beneath the nails, weight gain, etc. The expectant mother may not be aware of her diabetic condition, and she might consider these symptoms a side-effect of her pregnancy. Hence, it is always advisable to get yourself checked for Gestational Diabetes.

The uncontrolled sugar level might make your baby big, thereby leading to preterm labor. So, it is essential to monitor the sugar level in your blood closely. Unlike the previous ultrasound scans, this is a time where you could opt for a 3-D or 4-D scan of your baby.

The sixth month is a milestone for the baby. Hence, if you take a 3-D or 4-D scan, you could get a much closer look at your baby. I remember meeting a pregnant woman named Ananya, who came for a 3-D scan of the baby during her sixth month. While I was doing the scan, she asked me whether I could clearly show the baby's nose. I was curious and asked her the reason behind her question. She replied that her grandmother had Oriental facial features, and hence, she was afraid that the baby's nose might resemble hers.

The 3-D scan will help you see the baby's face clearly. I have encountered many such cases where women always wish to ensure that their baby does not possess certain traits of the family members, including baldness, or sharp or flat noses.

This is also a time for you to undertake a fetal echocardiogram. This is an ultrasound scan that helps check the baby's heart. If you have any history of heart issues in the family, it is advisable to take this scan to rule out the possibilities of such problems in the baby.

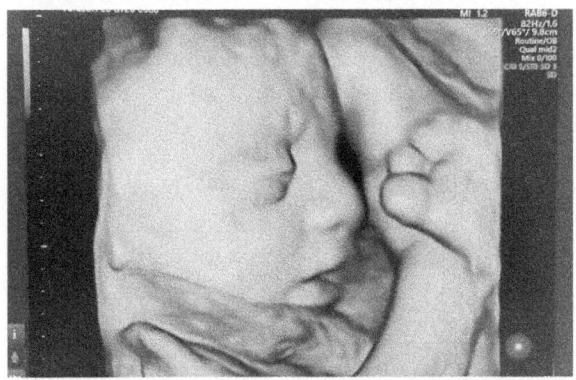

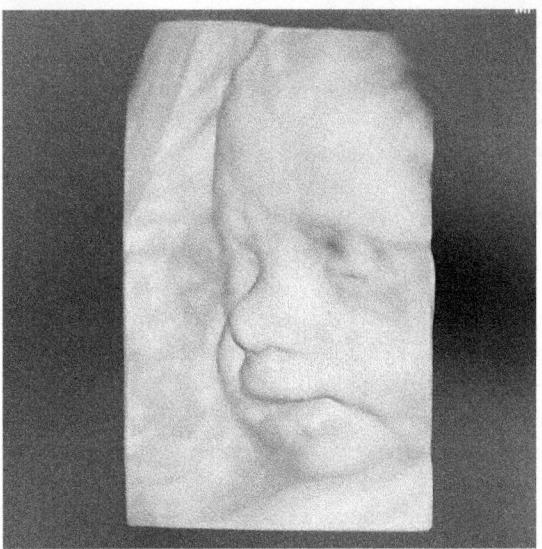

3-D Ultrasound Scan of the baby

The Doctor will also prescribe fetal echo if you have gestational Diabetes or the baby's heart structure is not properly visible during the anomaly scan. The baby's senses also develop during this phase. This is visible when the baby sucks its thumb during the scanning session.

A first-time mother-to-be who had come in for a scan once asked me who taught the babies to suck the breast milk. Sucking is a process that is learned by the baby even before it is born. It is an involuntary activity that starts from the womb itself; this signifies that the baby has matured taste buds. However, you might need to guide them in stopping this habit once they grow up.

The discomforts you experience during pregnancy will vary in the sixth month. This month, the significant discomfort you experience will be a stuffy nose. Pregnant women are supposed to drink at least eight glasses of water every day. My wife consumed ginger ale during her first pregnancy as if she was drinking water, which created worse scenarios. When she reached her sixth month, she started experiencing nasal congestion, which she attributed to the over-consumption of ginger ale. Ginger ale is an anti-inflammatory drink that soothes most of the discomforts you experience during pregnancy.

The nasal congestion you might experience is the by-product of pregnancy rhinitis, an inflammation of the mucous membranes lining the nose. Convincing your wife, especially a pregnant wife, is difficult, and hence I informed her about cutting down on ginger ale to get relief from nasal congestion.

One of my acquaintances commented that his wife wanted to see a dentist after delivery to put braces on her teeth as she always sleeps with her mouth open. She believed that this action was due to an elevation in the position of the teeth, which might wipe away her beauty.

He requested me to convince her as a Doctor. I shared my experience of the ginger ale with him, and he decided to meet the dentist soon after the delivery as he understood my situation!

Another troubling event during the sixth month is the Braxton-Hicks contraction. It is the body's tactics to prepare you for actual labor. Many women mistake Braxton-Hicks contraction to be a real one. A friend of mine took his wife to the hospital six times in the sixth month. Every time she experienced a contraction, she panicked and urged her husband to take her to the hospital.

At last, her Obstetrician suggested that she get admitted to the hospital for the next three months to avoid any further panic. Even though you might see the situation as funny, it is a prevalent phase that all pregnant women go through. Differentiating actual labor from false labor is a tiresome process.

Let me give you some tips on how to distinguish between actual labor and false labor. When you experience the contraction, you should check the time gap between each of them. False contractions are always irregular, whereas true contractions will be regular and get shorter as time passes. Likewise, when you experience pain and contraction, make sure to change your position. False contractions stop when you change the position.

However, true contractions will continue even if you change your positions or movements. I hope this chapter has given you ample insights into what to expect when you are six months pregnant.

Always remember one thing—the symptoms or discomforts vary from pregnancy-to-pregnancy and from one woman to another. Be prepared for the changes and discomforts because it is nature's way of molding you into the best mother. In the next chapter, let us take a detailed analysis of the seventh month.

23

PREGNANCY CALENDAR: SEVENTH MONTH

If you have entered the seventh month, that means you have completed two-thirds of your pregnancy journey. The seventh month marks the beginning of the third trimester or the last trimester. Ruby was a patient who consulted me for a 3-D ultrasound scan in her seventh month. She was a regular client who visited the clinic throughout her pregnancy and was very cheerful.

However, she was very gloomy when she approached me for the 3-D scan. I could see that she was feeling a bit low, and I enquired about the reason. She cried and said, "Doctor, I only have three more months for the delivery. I will miss the fantastic food and comforts that I received from everyone around me. Once the baby is born, everyone will be concerned about the baby alone and might scold me if I am not a good mother."

I was not surprised at her response, but I did feel sad for her. In my experience, I have seen many women like Ruby. If you are someone with the same feelings, do not blame yourself. This thought process is very normal as you approach the end of your pregnancy. The seventh month spans from the 28th week and goes on till the 31st week. Your uterus will enlarge itself to accommodate the growing baby.

The baby bump will be visible by this time, and you might be surprised to see the changes in the behavior of people around you. As the uterus grows, you might feel breathless and find it difficult to do many of your daily tasks.

For example, tying your shoelaces might feel like tying a leash around a restless dog. When my wife was pregnant for the first time, her Obstetrician ordered her to walk for at least half an hour every morning. However, our exercise session lasted more than 50 minutes, out of which tying the shoelaces took up more than 15 minutes. She never allowed me to help her with the laces; she also used to deny my help during our exercise sessions.

One of my friends mentioned his wife's inability to wash the dishes as her growing abdomen restricted her from reaching the kitchen pipe. Such discomforts will be part and parcel of your life as the growing baby demands more rest from the expectant mother's side. You might be tense about the development of the baby within your womb.

In the seventh month, your baby has many milestones to accomplish. This includes the development of facial features such as eyebrows, eyelashes, hair on the head, etc. Apart from that, this phase enables the baby to accumulate fat in its body in a very rampant manner. That is why Doctors suggest that the parents-to-be undertake the 3-D scan in the sixth or the seventh month. Another milestone that the baby accomplishes this month is the development of footprints and fingerprints. Indeed, the seventh month is a starting point for the maturation of the baby's many internal and external organs.

Hence, if an emergency occurs and the baby has to be taken out, it has a 90 percent chance of survival with good ICU and neonatal care facilities. Many babies start to open and close their eyes during this phase, enabling the baby to regularize its sleeping pattern. Once the sleeping pattern is regularized, it will be easy for the mother-to-be to check for the baby's movements.

I remember meeting Shyla, a seven-month pregnant woman who complained of absent baby movements. She was unaware of the sleeping pattern and was worried when she could not feel the baby's kicks. When she was in the hospital's emergency section, she complained about the issue at hand and sought help. Her Obstetrician immediately gave her some sugar. After she consumed the sugar, she experienced the baby's kick again.

There are many instances like this that I have heard of and encountered myself. When the baby starts following a sleep pattern, you might not experience the baby's kicks during its sleep. It would help if you learned to track the sleep pattern so that an absence of the baby's kick during its sleep will not panic you.

If you cannot feel the baby during its usual active time, you should consume some sweet substance to rouse the baby from sleep. Most Obstetricians inform you to check for the baby's movement once or twice a day, 15 or 20 minutes after the major meals.

HOW TO COUNT BABY KICKS?

Counting is done in a lying down position or sitting position. Count all the baby movements, including soft swishes, until you reach 10 counts. Normally, there should be 10 counts in one hour. If the count is less than 10 in an hour, eat something and then recount. If the baby's kicks are weak, or if you could not feel the baby even after consuming food or sweet substances, you should immediately inform your Obstetrician.

A friend of mine mentioned that he took his wife five times during her seventh month as she could not feel the baby's movements. However, before reaching the hospital, the baby's kick became prominent. Then onwards, whenever his wife complained of the absence of the baby's kick, he used to take her for a ride, after which the baby's kick was felt. I still did not know the baby kicked during the ride and not before that! My wife always asked me to experience this blissful kick by putting my hand over her belly.

In the seventh month and the eighth month, I could not experience it. By the time she was near her delivery date, I could see the baby's foot on her belly as the kicks became solid and prominent. The baby's kick you experience in the seventh month might resemble false labor pain, and you might feel as if the baby is coming out at that instance. Unless the pain is accompanied by vaginal bleeding or vomiting, there is no need to panic. By the time you are seven months pregnant, your baby will weigh around 1.4 kg and be 10 inches long. I recall meeting Rudra, a pregnant woman who had to undergo a C-Section as she developed pre-eclampsia in the seventh month.

Her baby was so tiny and was placed in the incubator for proper growth and nourishment. Her husband, Manoj, who got a chance to see the baby in the incubator, came out and announced to the relatives that the baby was as tiny as a newborn kitten. I was passing through the neonatal ICU's dormitory and was surprised to hear Manoj's comment. I had never heard such a comparison before in my life.

I inquired about the case with a nurse who was standing there. I later shared this incident with my wife. She reminded me that Manoj, as a farmer, could only compare the size of the baby with something he was familiar with, a kitten. My wife said, "You cannot expect him to compare the size of the baby with something from the medical or scientific world. Well, as he is familiar with animals and farming, he compared the size of the baby with that of a kitten".

When we reflect on the mother's uterus, we find its size increases along with its height. The uterus will acquire a position between the naval and the breast. Hence, many women will encounter a popping out of the belly button. I had a pregnant patient who refused to exhibit her baby tummy as her belly button had popped out. She was seven months pregnant and was asked to take an ultrasound scan to check for a hernia. It took me nearly fifteen minutes to make her realize that the popped-out belly button was normal during pregnancy.

Nausea that would have vanished during the second trimester might reappear during the third trimester. The growing uterus will exert pressure on all the other organs in the body, including the stomach and intestines. You may feel a kind of ***heaviness in the chest and the abdomen***. Many women complain of heartburn and chest heaviness during this phase and worry about heart issues. Breathlessness, heaviness, etc., are symptoms of pregnancy that could be attributed to the growing uterus. If you feel unable to breathe correctly after taking a few steps, do not blame your weight. It is not your weight; instead, the uterus making space to accommodate the baby is the real culprit. You might have heard the maxim "slow and steady wins the race". It is better to uphold this maxim in the third trimester than work faster and get exhausted very soon. Another major discomfort you might experience during this phase is the ***Braxton Hicks contraction***. Some women mistake it to be real contractions and will rush to the hospital fearing preterm labor.

During this phase, you might experience constipation, which results from the pressure of the uterus on the intestines. **Constipation** is something you should be very careful about during this phase. When you feel constipated, you will exert pressure to pass the stools. When excessive force is used, that might result in preterm delivery. If a pregnant woman suffers from constipation issues, the Doctor might prescribe stool softening medicines or homemade remedies to avoid preterm labor conditions. **Sciatic pain** is another troubling discomfort you might experience during this phase. It is a pain you feel in the lower back, which will radiate toward the back of the leg.

A hot pad or bed rest will help you get relief from the pain. You might also experience *oily secretions around your nipple*, which is the body's natural way of preparing your breasts for breastfeeding. A sudden hike in fatigue is another feature that you should be aware of in the seventh month. To accomplish the milestones, the baby within you will suck up the nutrient components present in the body in a very high amount. This will result in severe tiredness. If you are not following a healthy diet, then the third trimester will be a big hurdle. The uterus's pressure will also be felt on the urinary bladder, releasing urine in dribbles involuntarily.

From this week onwards, the mother will gain 500 gm of weight every week. Never try to reduce your food intake due to the increase in weight. It is not fat accumulation that causes a sudden increase in weight; instead, it is the growth of the uterus and placenta that results in a sudden increase in body weight.

I met a pregnant woman named Shylaja, who was admitted because of severe dizziness. As Shylaja had gained weight, she cut down her food intake hoping for a normal delivery. However, this action resulted in a drop of nutrients in her body. She had to stay in the hospital for more than a week to recover.

During her stay, the Doctors gave a clear lecture on being prepared for pregnancy and the changes during and after pregnancy. She was studying for undergraduate degree when she got pregnant. Later, I learnt that she took up a dietician course for her master's degree and is currently working as a pregnancy dietician in the hospital where she was admitted.

In your seventh month, the first and foremost thing you should do is sit back and relax. A renowned phase of discomfort is approaching, followed by a long tenure of the active phase.

The following two months will bring more pains than what you are experiencing now, and once the delivery is over, you would have to start adjusting your timings with that of the newborn. I remember a friend of mine did not get enough time to sleep in the first three months after her delivery. She commented that "the baby was supposed to be born in America, but was accidentally born in India". It took three months for the baby to regularize its sleeping pattern.

On the other hand, another friend of mine created a sleeping atmosphere for the baby; the baby fell asleep in that environment. There was a minor issue with this sleeping practice because when they moved to another place, the baby refused to sleep as she needed the sleeping atmosphere to which she was accustomed.

Your Doctor might advise you to have regular check-ups twice a week from the seventh month onwards, especially if you have a high-risk pregnancy. It is mandatory to follow the Doctor's advice, as any failure might create complications for you and your baby. I once met a couple who were not up-to-date with their check-ups. Hence, they did not follow much of the instructions provided by their medical care specialist. The mother-to-be developed gestational Diabetes in the sixth month. Hence, an emergency C-Section was conducted to deliver the baby boy who was more than 3 kg in his seventh month. The baby survived as the hospital had good neonatal facilities, but it took more than a year to get the baby to a routine as he had suffered trauma during the procedure. It is better to listen to the Doctor rather than ending up with severe complications.

This is a phase when the baby sets into a position—the head down position. Baby movements become more intense due to the availability of more space in the uterus, and hence, they often respond to various stimuli like external sounds, light, and the food you consume. It is also a phase where your baby starts sucking its thumb. Did you know that babies get dreams while they are inside your womb? You read it right. The recorded brain wave activity shows rapid eye movements at this stage, when dreaming occurs.

Boostrix is a vaccine that most pregnant women take during the seventh month of pregnancy. It boosts the immune systems of the mothers-to-be and prevents them from contracting whooping cough, diphtheria, and tetanus. In the next chapter, let us quickly check what to expect when you enter the eighth month.

24

PREGNANCY CALENDAR: EIGHTH MONTH

I was reading some notes on pregnancy and happened to find a very inspiring quote by an anonymous writer. It said, "Some of the days you feel so inadequate that you might not be strong enough to be a mother, then there's a lively kick inside you, and it reminds you there's someone who already believes in you." If you have not experienced strong punches yet, be ready for surprises because once you enter your eighth month, the boxer inside you is all equipped for a tough fight. The eighth month spans from the 32nd week to the 35th week.

I will never forget Krithi, a pregnant woman who complained about such changes to my wife when they met at the Doctor's clinic. My wife was two months pregnant at that time and was coming to meet her Doctor for the first time. She was anxious, and, at the same time, excited about being a first-time mother. Kriti, on the other hand, had come for her eighth-month check-up. Her tummy was so huge that anyone who saw it would immediately think that she was carrying more than one baby. My wife, too, felt the same and asked Kriti if she was carrying twins or triplets. Kriti, however, replied that it wasn't a multiple pregnancy; she appeared to be irritated by her large tummy. Being a Doctor, I decided to give Kriti some advice.

When I informed her about the possible changes during this phase, she asked me if I was an Obstetrician to have first-hand knowledge about these issues. I replied that I was a Fetal Radiologist who had at least second-hand knowledge about pregnancy.

Do you know why I am talking about Kriti here? It is to pinpoint that the mental, physical and emotional changes you experience during this phase might create an imbalance in your relationship with others. You might attribute this imbalance to mood changes.

You might develop new anxiety, known as "nearing due date" anxiety, during this phase. I remember meeting Arathi, a pregnant patient from Kerala. She had cervical incompetence initially, and hence the Doctors put a suture on the cervical opening. Once she completed her 30th week, the Doctors removed the suture. Within the next three weeks, she visited the hospital five times, complaining about contractions.

Her Doctors realized that the patient suffered from anxiety and decided to provide a counseling session for her. During the counseling session, she revealed that she was tensed about the gender of the baby. She was also concerned about the pain she had to endure during the delivery. After a few sittings, we addressed her anxieties, and I did not see her in the hospital until her delivery date. Being anxious is a normal condition during pregnancy. However, getting a counseling session is crucial if it affects your daily life or leads to unwanted worries and thoughts.

A friend of mine working in a hospital in Trivandrum mentioned a similar case where a woman accidentally consumed some wrong medicines due to a higher degree of anxiety. Instead of pain medication, she consumed medicine that is used to lower sugar levels. Her sugar level went down, and she was immediately taken to the hospital.

Later, it was revealed that she had been suffering from anxiety as her due date was near. Some of the significant discomforts you might experience during this phase include pelvic pressure, leg cramps, back pain, swollen ankle, hemorrhoids, etc. My wife, during her first pregnancy, used to complain about leg cramps.

One night she had severe leg cramps, and she jumped out of bed. I was worried and told her never to repeat this action, as a sudden jump might sometimes cause complications. It is believed that muscle cramps or leg cramps occur due to insufficient blood circulation to the legs.

Hence, make it a point to do some activities with the legs so that you can avoid these types of cramping issues to a certain level. You might wonder and feel proud about the sudden growth of your hair. A patient who came to me for an ultrasound scan commented that she could enact the role of Rapunzel, but with her enlarged stomach, she might not be able to pull the prince up to the tower! You should thank the pregnancy hormones for these sudden changes in your hair quality and quantity. You might experience hair fall with the delivery as the pregnancy hormones will no longer be present in your body.

I recall meeting Savitha, who was taken into the emergency department as she experienced chest pain and breathlessness during the eighth month of pregnancy. As only the juniors were present in the emergency, I was informed to look at the case, as she was pregnant. Her ECG was normal, and those at the emergency department were planning to send for an ECHO. I decided to talk with her family before consenting to the procedure. I wanted to re-check if ECHO was necessary or not. I realized after my conversation that she was doing her pregnancy exercises and immediately felt a sharp pain in the chest, accompanied by breathlessness. However, we decided to conduct the ECHO as she mentioned chest pain again. The ECHO result was also normal, and hence I thought of having a conversation with her. She was hyperventilating when I approached her, and the Doctors in charge were giving her oxygen. I sat beside her, and after a few minutes, her breathing pattern became normal. Even before I could ask anything, she mentioned the exercise, the sudden pain, and the tension she experienced that led to hyperventilation. I was taken aback when I heard her using so many medical terms during the conversation. She was an MBBS student who was currently doing her house surgency. Due to the strenuous work schedule and the pregnancy, she was tensed. The pressure exerted on the ribs by the growing uterus added to the pain. Before she could explain the situation, her husband took her back home. I then met her husband, who was unaware of all these changes that were happening to her body. This incident was an eye-opener for me. Many husbands, except those from the medical field, are unaware of the changes happening to their partners during pregnancy. From then onwards, I made it a point to give clear counseling sessions to the father-to-be to help them understand their partner's strain.

One of my friends, during our reunion, commented that his wife is a spider woman now. The phrase 'spider woman' was a disturbing one as we all knew that she was carrying their fourth child. I called him aside and asked him why he used that phrase to describe his wife. He was not teasing her, but was being sympathetic for her current issue.

She had so many spider-like blue markings on her body. You might have noticed such markings on your body, especially around your thighs and legs. These spider-like discolorations that you find on your body are varicose veins formed as the veins beneath your skin get engorged. These are not permanent markings and will disappear with the delivery. Varicose veins that appear in the anal area create itching and pain while passing stool. If you have similar experiences, you should inform this problem to your medical practitioner, who will prescribe medicines as well as home remedies to get rid of the discomforts associated with it.

You might also experience a need to change your innerwear, especially your bra, as your breast enlarges. The prolactin and other milk-producing hormones are ready for the big day when you start breastfeeding. You might experience a feeling of fullness that might create discomfort for you.

I had a celebrity patient who had come for her 3-D scan. She was more concerned about her enlarged tummy and breasts and asked me several times whether it would come back to normal once the pregnancy was over. I affirmed that the abdomen would become normal after delivery, provided that she put in enough effort. However, I could not promise her that the breasts could go back to their regular size as the mother needs to breastfeed the child. Many women wish to recover their original beauty and body qualities after their delivery. Some women achieve it with rigorous exercise and a strict diet, whereas others may not achieve this target. I have seen many women pondering their lost beauty by comparing their previous pictures with their current ones. If you are one among them, do not feel sad. Remember that an outstanding achievement comes with many sacrifices and struggles, and I firmly believe that being a mother is such an accomplishment.

The eighth month is notable for experiencing false labor, which many women mistake for actual labor. I have already mentioned many cases in which women mistook false labor for the true one and rushed to the hospital in a panic mode.

Uterine contractions are a common phenomenon during this phase. Hence, it is vital to understand how to differentiate actual labor from a false one. The table given below will help you to distinguish between actual labor and false labor.

TRUE LABOUR	FALSE LABOUR
Contractions come at regular intervals and get closer as time passes.	Contractions are not regular.
Contractions continue even with a position change or movements.	Contractions might stop with a position change or movement.

You should be aware of the symptoms of preterm labor during this phase. There is a chance of preterm labor as the pregnancy progresses, especially if you previously had preterm delivery. It would help if you watched out for symptoms such as tightness in the lower abdomen, heaviness in the lower abdomen and thighs, fluid leakage, spotting or mild bleeding from the vagina, and at least six consecutive contractions within one hour that are 10 minutes apart. Inform your medical practitioner about these issues and move to the hospital as soon as possible.

Itchiness and dry skin will be another aggravating factor you might experience during pregnancy, especially in the eighth and ninth months. The more you scratch, the more markings appear on your body. The growing uterus causes the skin to stretch, and this stretching is the primary cause of this itchiness. It is believed that at least 20 percent of pregnant women experience this irritating effect. Sometimes, this can also be a symptom of an underlying liver problem. Hence, your Doctor might suggest you undergo a liver function test and liver ultrasound scan.

Finding a comfortable sleeping position will be a tricky thing to achieve during this phase. Due to the enlarged abdomen, Doctors suggest you to sleep on your sides. However, sleeping on the sides also needs to be tailored appropriately according to your comfortable position. To achieve this milestone, you could use a sleeping pillow to support your tummy.

It can also be kept between your thighs for acquiring the perfect sleeping position. Usually, during this phase, your Doctors will inform you to visit them every week until the delivery to observe the changes happening to you and your baby. It is crucial to attend these check-ups without any delay as negligence might trigger pregnancy issues. If you have any doubts regarding cord-blood banking, this is the right time to discuss this with your Doctor.

I have already mentioned about this in a separate chapter in the later part of the book. I have been talking about the discomforts and specific topics that you might encounter during your eighth month. Now, let us have a close look at the developmental milestones of your baby.

Till now, the weight of the baby was increasing at a slow pace. However, the eighth month marks the drastic and sudden weight gain of the child. It is scientifically proven that during this month, babies gain about 250–300 gm every week. The sleep–wake cycle is almost fixed by this time, and the mother will distinguish this timing properly. This is also a phase where the baby will develop breathing movements called hiccups. The hiccups can be easily distinguished as it creates periodic twitches or spasms over the mother's tummy. By the time you complete your eighth month, the baby will be around 15–18 inch long and weigh about 1.5–2.5 kg.

The baby's movements will be reduced during this phase, and hence if you feel less intense kicks, do not panic. This is mainly due to reduced space in the uterus as the baby within you is growing. Even though the lungs of the baby are almost developed, they are not yet fully functional. The baby's digestive system will be fully developed by this time. Even though most babies are set down to the head-down position, nearly five percent of babies will settle at being in the bottom-down or breech position. During the scans, many women enquire about the position of the baby. If they realize that the baby is bottom-down, the next question that I often encounter is whether there is any chance for the baby to flip down. Remember that babies might flip later, especially if there is enough liquor volume (fluid) and space within the uterus.

The eighth month is a good phase for the mother to rest. As the baby's growth is rapid, mothers are often advised to take rest to fight against fatigue and tiredness. If your Obstetrician anticipates a preterm delivery, they will advise for an intramuscular steroid injection that would help to mature the baby's lungs faster.

I recall one such case that I encountered in one of the leading hospitals in Trivandrum. The mother, Reeba, had placenta previa, and she was in her eighth month. After discussing the case with other Doctors, I reported the issue to her Obstetrician, who recommended a C-section delivery. They decided to give two injections of Betamethasone 24 hours apart.

All this information was conveyed to Reeba's husband, who disagreed with the Betamethasone injection. The junior Doctor did not inform him that the steroid was meant to mature the baby's lungs. When he heard the term steroid, he started an argument with the junior Doctor stating that steroids were harmful during pregnancy. However, as the argument became strong, the senior Doctor revealed the true intention behind administering the injection. She was taken into the operating room after being administered the two doses. She gave birth to a baby girl, whom the parents named Soney, after the steroid's name.

I hope this chapter has provided ample input on what to expect when you are in the eighth month. Now, let us move on to the changes that could be expected in the ninth month in the next chapter.

25

PREGNANCY CALENDAR: NINTH MONTH

The weeks that range from the 36th to the 40th comprise the ninth month of pregnancy. Entering the ninth month is a giant leap as the baby born after this period has a high chance of survival, sometimes even without the aid of an incubator. The baby is fully developed by the 37th week. I recall meeting Shantha, who complained about contractions and was admitted to the hospital. Even though she was experiencing real labor pain, her cervix was not dilating.

The Doctors waited for more than 12 hours, but as the cervix was not dilated enough, they decided to take the baby out through a C-section. I was called to conduct an ultrasound scan to check for the baby's position and the placenta. While undertaking the scan, I realized that the baby was more than 4 kg in weight. So, normal delivery would have been tough. I informed the Doctors, who then decided to deliver the baby through C-section.

However, when they told Shantha about their decision, she begged them to give her two more hours, as she wanted a normal delivery. After discussing with the seniors and the other Doctors, her Obstetrician allowed her to wait for two more hours. After this allotted time, they were planning to take her to the operation theatre.

I do not know what miracle she performed, but after half an hour, when the Doctors checked her cervix, it was 8 cm dilated. They waited for a couple of minutes, and she was ready for the delivery within no time.

After the procedure, I met her and inquired about this miracle. When the Doctor had informed her about the C-section procedure, Shantha decided to walk around a bit; that is all. All those attending to her in the labor room were surprised to experience this miracle.

Usually, it is challenging to have a normal delivery if the baby is above 3.5 kg or 4 kg. However, in the case of Shantha, vaginal delivery was possible. By the time you complete your 35th week, the baby's lungs will be thoroughly developed. Despite that, if the baby is born before the 35th week, it is called early preterm, and if the baby is born between the 35th to 37th weeks, it is called late preterm. In both these cases, ICU care is needed depending upon the baby's breathing condition and oxygen saturation. That is why birth centers should have ICU and neonatal care facilities.

I remember my friend mentioning "The Mythri" case, where a pregnant woman named Mythri gave birth to a baby in the 36th week. The baby had birth trauma and needed special care in the ICU. However, the birth center that the parents chose had no neonatal ICU facility. Hence, the father took the baby to another hospital that had an ICU facility.

The mother was admitted to the previous birth center as she had some bleeding issues. The mother could not feed the baby for the next five days, which led to many discomforts. After five days, she went to the other hospital to feed the baby when she got discharged. My friend mentioned that Mythri's case was not a rarity. Many people are ignorant about the need for neonatal services in the hospital they choose for delivery.

During the ninth month, you will experience different types of movements within your womb, similar to rolls, stretches, and wiggles. Your baby cannot properly move as it is cramped in the small space within your womb.

You might feel irritated when you realize that your baby is disturbing your peaceful sleep patterns. I had a patient named Ammu, who complained about insomnia as her baby was moving at night. Her mother consoled her and told her that it would be okay once the baby was born. Six months after her delivery, she came to meet me for an ultrasound scan.

Out of curiosity, I asked her whether she was getting enough sleep now, to which she laughed out loud in response. She commented that her baby had just started maintaining a good sleep pattern. Till that time, the baby used to wake up every hour at night demanding to be fed. This is not a case unique to Ammu. Many pregnant women have similar experiences. After all, motherhood is synonymous with sacrifice, which also includes sacrificing your peaceful sleep pattern.

You will experience severe tiredness during this month. The baby inside your womb will be doing all the final preparations before the big day. Your baby will use up all the nutrients you have stored in your body from the different food and supplements you consumed in preparation for this time. If you are familiar with "the hare and the tortoise" story, then this will be the right time to follow the maxim proposed by the story, that is, "slow and steady wins the race". During this phase, it is advisable to slow down and relax as the baby needs more care on your part. Like severe tiredness, another discomfort that might bother you during this phase will be shortness of breath.

I remember my wife struggling with this issue during her ninth month. Whenever you wish to move or walk, you will be held back due to the shortness of breath you experience. Sometimes, this is a blessing in disguise. I encountered a patient named Rema who had a minor accident during her ninth month. She was working in the kitchen and heard her mobile ringing in the other room. As she was walking to get the phone, she slipped on some water on the floor and fell down. She prayed that her baby was safe throughout the scanning procedure; she later mentioned that her condition would have probably been critical if she had run faster. She also commented that it was the shortness of breath that made her unable to run fast. Most women will experience a sense of absent-mindedness or panic during this phase, leading to complications if left unchecked. Shortness of breath is a controlling factor that puts a halt to potential accidents. The baby settles in one position during this month, enabling the Obstetrician to decide on the type of delivery that could happen. There are mainly three common fetal positions in the uterus—cephalic, breech, and transverse positions. The cephalic position is the ideal position for normal delivery. Here, "the baby is positioned head down, facing your back, with the chin tucked to its chest and the back of the head ready to enter the pelvis."

By the end of the ninth month, most babies settle to one of these positions.

The baby's buttocks will be near the cervix in the breech position, and in the occiput posterior position, the baby's face will be up. I have encountered numerous would-be parents who ask whether there is a chance for normal delivery? There are so many factors that determine the mode of delivery, and a Radiologist will not have the power to predict it. It is complicated to attempt a vaginal birth if the baby is in a breech position because the child's head might get trapped in the cervix during the procedure. Sometimes your healthcare provider might try to turn the baby before the onset of labor. This might not happen properly in some cases, which ultimately results in a C-section delivery.

You might also experience quickening this month, which is a relief felt in the upper abdomen when the baby drops down. Some may experience the quickening process a few weeks before the actual labor, whereas others experience it with the starting of labor. Hence, do not mistake quickening as a sign of the beginning of labor.

I remember Kareena, who came for her ultrasound scan in the ninth month. The baby was in the cephalic position, and everything about the baby was normal. I told her not to be worried as the baby was fine. Soon after my comment, she asked me whether the baby's head was fixed in the pelvis. The baby had not dropped down to the pelvis, and hence I informed her that it would only happen with the onset of pregnancy. Many mothers-to-be have the same doubt as they are doubtful whether their babies are struggling to get oxygen. Always remember that the baby's head will only get fixed during active labor.

As the baby grows, you will feel extra pressure on the urinary bladder, making you urinate more often at night. I happened to meet Riya, a nine-month pregnant woman who was admitted to a hospital in Bangalore. I was her Radiologist throughout her pregnancy, and hence the hospital authorities requested me to conduct her ultrasound scan. She was admitted due to a urinary tract infection (UTI), and having an UTI in the ninth month is not a good sign, as per the Obstetricians.

As she was pretty familiar to me, I asked her if she was drinking the right amount of water. She revealed that to avoid multiple visits to the bathroom at night and experience good sleep, she had reduced her water intake at night.

This practice is a wrong method that pregnant women sometimes adopt. Reducing water intake and skipping bathroom visits amidst an urge to urinate result in UTI, which, left untreated, might affect the health of the baby and the mother-to-be. The ninth month is the right time to start Kegel exercises. This exercise will help to improve the tone of the muscles surrounding the pelvic region that support the uterus and the urinary bladder. It also helps tone up the pelvic floor so that the discomfort you might experience during the ninth and the tenth months can be reduced to a large extent. Regular pelvic exercises will help reduce pelvic floor injuries that may occur during the delivery. Nipple discharge is another common symptom experienced during the ninth month.

I remember Ananya, a pregnant woman who came for a mammogram test during her pregnancy. She complained about nipple discharge, and her Obstetrician tried to educate her about the symptoms she would experience during her ninth month. Despite listening to a series of lectures on nipple discharge, she continued to complain, fearing that she would not be able to feed her baby. Hence, at last, her Obstetrician decided to let her undertake a mammogram to convince her that nipple discharge was common during pregnancy. After the test, I conveyed that everything was normal and that nipple discharge was acceptable during pregnancy. I experienced a heart-touching appreciation for the service I provided.

I did not do anything magical there. My findings were similar to that of the Obstetrician. However, she acted like St. Thomas, who asked for evidence to believe the resurrection of Christ. With the evidence I provided through the mammogram result, she believed me. Even though that was a heart-warming incident, I told her to trust her Obstetrician rather than waiting for shreds of evidence.

Many birthing centers offer counseling sessions for would-be parents. Enrolling yourself in these sessions is preferable as they will prepare you to face the different labor and delivery processes. Your Doctor will schedule appointments every week to evaluate the progress of your pregnancy. Along with that, they will inform you to check for labor symptoms such as regular contractions, leakage of amniotic fluid from the vagina, vaginal bleeding, and so on. It is crucial to check for the presence of these symptoms during pregnancy. Your Obstetrician will also perform a pelvic or vaginal examination to check the cervix for softening and dilation.

SYMPTOMS OF TRUE LABOUR
• Regular contractions at regular intervals • Leakage of vaginal fluid • Vaginal bleeding • Sharp pain in the pelvic area accompanied by spotting or bleeding • Mucus discharge, especially blood-colored • Severe pain in the belly and lower back

An ultrasound scan is usually advised during the ninth month. This helps in understanding the position and weight of the baby, the quantity of the amniotic fluid, and the position of the placenta. Scanning also helps in assessing the blood flow to the baby and detecting whether the cord is around the baby neck. You should also make it a point to go through the birth plan checklist and be ready with all the items needed before, during, and after the delivery.

DELIVERY CHECK-LIST
• Hospital File, ID card, insurance papers • Dressing gown/Feeding nighty • Socks • Slippers • Massage oil • Comfortable Pillows • Relaxing pass-times (books, mobile phone) • Heavy duty maternity pads • Disposable inner wears • Toiletries • Newborn wear: socks, booties, blankets, diapers, dresses, etc.

Let us quickly summarize the baby's development in all the three trimesters before proceeding with the other topics associated with pregnancy.

26

MILESTONES ACCOMPLISHED AT EVERY MONTH

Pregnancy is a journey that lasts for nearly nine months. One of the major anxieties that pregnant women often have is their baby's well-being. Many pregnant women often ask about the baby's height, weight, etc. I encountered similar questions from my wife when she was carrying our first daughter. Hence, in this chapter, I wish to provide an insight into the baby's development week-wise.

In the table on the next page, I have attempted to compare the baby's size at different weeks of pregnancy with common objects that are familiar to us; this will give you ample knowledge about your baby's size, length, and weight.

Week	Size of the Baby	Length of the Baby	Weight of the Baby
One and Two (Menstruation and Pre-ovulatory period)	No visible pregnancy		
Three (Ovulation and Fertilization)			
Four (Implantation)	Like a poppy seed	Less than 1 mm	
Five	Size of an orange seed		
Six	Size of a sweet pea	0.51-0.64 cm	
Seven	Size of a blueberry	0.64 cm	
Eight	Size of a raspberry	1.27 cm	
Nine	Size of a green olive	2.54 cm	
Ten	Size of a prune	3-4 cm	
Eleven	Size of a strawberry	4 cm	7 gm
Twelve	Size of a lime	5-6 cm	14 gm
Thirteen	Size of a big lime	8 cm	28 gm
Fourteen	Size of a navel orange	9-10 cm	57 gm

DUE DATE

Fifteen	Size of a pear	10 cm	71 gm
Sixteen	Size of an avocado	10-13 cm	0.11 kg
Seventeen	Size of a large onion	13 cm	0.14 kg
Eighteen	Size of a cucumber	14 cm	0.14-0.18 kg
Nineteen	Size of a mango	15 cm	0.23 kg
Twenty	Size of a sweet potato	16.5 cm	0.28 kg
Twenty-one	Size of a big banana	27 cm	0.31-0.35 kg
Twenty-two	Size of a bell pepper	28 cm	0.45 kg
Twenty-three	Size of a big grapefruit	28 cm	0.54 kg
Twenty-four	Size of a big pomegranate	29 cm	0.59 kg
Twenty-five	Size of an eggplant	33 cm	0.68 kg
Twenty-six	Size of an acorn squash	36 cm	0.91 kg
Twenty-seven	Size of a cabbage	37 cm	0.91 kg
Twenty-eight	Size of a lettuce	38 cm	1 kg

Twenty-nine	Size of a cauliflower	39-41 cm	1.1-1.4 kg
Thirty	Size of a bunch of broccoli	41 cm	1.4 kg
Thirty-one	Size of a big coconut	41 cm	1.5 kg
Thirty-two	Size of a cantaloupe	41-43 cm	1.6-1.8 kg
Thirty-three	Size of a butternut squash	43 cm	1.9 kg
Thirty-four	Size of a pineapple	43-46 cm	2.3 kg
Thirty-five	Size of a spaghetti squash	46 cm	2.4 kg
Thirty-six	Size of a bunch of kale	46-48 cm	2.7 kg
Thirty-seven	Size of a canary melon	48 cm	2.9 kg
Thirty-eight	Size of a mini watermelon	48-51 cm	3.2 kg
Thirty-nine	Size of a honeydew melon	48-53 cm	3.2-3.6 kg
Forty	Size of a small pumpkin	48-56 cm	3.2-4.1 kg

27

LABOR AND DELIVERY

The term "labor" can strike fear in many women. I have personally witnessed women who scream a lot while experiencing labor pain. Labor pain has been described as excruciating, and this is probably the most painful phase a woman experiences in her life. However, many people are unaware that this phase can be smoothed over if you are mentally relaxed.

In many cases, as soon as labor begins, the pregnant woman starts to panic. The two main reasons for this panic are ignorance of what happens during labor and concern about the baby yet to be born. The term labor means "work, especially physical work". The labor associated with pregnancy is also physical work that can be accomplished with full participation from your side. This is the phase where you put a full stop to the long wait, which could have lasted for nine months.

However, for certain people, this full stop arrives even before completion of the nine-month journey. I remember meeting a patient named Saraswathi, who was screaming in the pre-labor room. The labor had just started for her.

However, her cry was so loud that everyone around her thought that she had reached the last stage of labor. Finally, the Doctors decided to move her to a secluded space so that her panic screams would not frighten the other women.

I still recall Anitha, one of the other patients, who asked me if it was always so harrowing during labor. I smiled at her and replied that I was new to the department. I do not know whether she understood what I said; however, she did not ask me anything from then. Saraswati gave birth to a baby boy after going through prolonged labor. If she had been mentally prepared to relax a bit, the labor and delivery might have been smoother.

You might have decided on the hospital where you want to have your baby and the type of delivery you prefer by this time. However, you should maintain a mindset to change your options in case of an emergency. Most women prefer a normal vaginal delivery. There is a misconception regarding C-section delivery, that the pain and discomforts following it will last throughout life. Even though it is partly correct, proper rest and following the Doctor's advice will help to relieve the procedure's discomfort. It is essential to ask your Doctor about getting admitted to the hospital for the delivery.

It is vital to know that the labor experience varies from person to person. For instance, the pain you experience during your first delivery will be higher compared to that in subsequent deliveries. I remember meeting Natasha, who came for her third delivery, which was smooth. She suffered from pain for 10 minutes, and the baby arrived very quickly. When asked about her experience, she mentioned that she had experienced labor pains for more than six hours during her first delivery.

Hence, make it a point to engage in a counseling session with your Obstetrician, nursing assistant, and counselor to understand the labor procedure thoroughly. The more you know, the less panicked you will be. Once the fear of labor is gone, you will enjoy the process with excitement for the baby's arrival. Remember to complete the registration and insurance formalities beforehand. If you have not packed your hospital bag yet, then this is the right time for doing so. Be ready beforehand so that last-minute tensions or emergencies will not catch you unaware and make you forget to collect the bag that is most needed during and after the delivery.

While undergoing house surgency, we were supposed to meet the people who took charge of the different departments. I remember meeting a nurse who was in charge of the labor room. She shouted at the patient's family members for not bringing the dhoti or cotton sari, claiming that the patient will later complain of a lax abdomen if it is not appropriately bound soon after the delivery.

I recalled this incident, and when my wife packed her bag for delivery, I shared this incident with her; she revealed that she had purchased an abdominal binder for this purpose. Make it a point to discuss with your Obstetrician the items you need to carry with you when you get admitted for your delivery. Some hospitals provide baby accessories and maternity accessories. Hence, have an open discussion about this with your Doctor.

Your body will give specific signals to inform you about the approaching phase of labor. This includes lightening, the process in which the baby drops down to the pelvic area; bloody vaginal discharge; etc. Unlike the first-time mothers, the others might not feel lightening as it happens just before the onset of labor. However, first-time mothers might easily recognize lightning as the baby's dropping will allow them to breathe easier.

Many women have asked me about the bodily changes during labor and some of the terminologies Doctors used during their check-ups. If you have heard your Doctor saying "effacement", that means the cervix becomes thin. This is assessed during a physical examination, and the effacement is expressed in percentage. When the cervix is completely effaced, it is called 100 percent effaced. The next term you might hear is dilation. However, your cervix has to open from 0–10 cm to facilitate the baby's delivery

The cervix's dilation is also assessed during a physical examination, where your Doctor inserts her fingers inside the vagina to determine the measurement. A significant change that happens during labor is the breaking of water. Only a few women experience a sudden gush of water (amniotic fluid). In other cases, the water leaks, and you may be able to experience water leaking from the vagina.

Contractions are the next change you will experience as the labor progresses. Unlike Braxton-Hicks contractions, labor contractions will be regular and get stronger with time. If you experience the above-said signs, you should immediately move to the hospital as the baby is ready to be born. By this time, your Doctor will advise you on whom to call and when to report to the hospital. It is advisable to go to the hospital after an hour of the regular contractions. These contractions should happen at regular five-minute intervals. Sometimes the contractions may stop or reduce in intensity. In such a case, after observation and clinical assessment, you may be advised to go home and come back to the hospital after real labor sets in.

A friend of mine narrated her labor experiences to me. She was at her house when the pain started, which panicked her father and brothers. However, her mother, who had undergone labor four times, was calm and patient. She even mentioned that her mother took an extra 15 minutes to drape the saree, which she used to do within five minutes. Even after reaching the hospital, it took more than five hours for the baby to be born. Her mother would later comment that patience is required for labor. What she said is correct. If we have patience, we will relax, and this ultimately leads to a smooth delivery. On the other hand, impatience leads to tension and panic, paving the way for pregnancy complications. Labor is divided into three phases for the convenience of monitoring its progress.

The first stage: It involves progress from regular uterine contractions to partial opening of the cervix. This stage is the longest stage of labor, which can last for hours. I have seen many women walking around the pre-labor room to hasten this process as the baby's weight and constant walking might help speed up the cervix's dilation process.

The second stage: This is from the cervix's complete opening till the baby's delivery. This phase can last anywhere from 20 minutes to hours. As far as the pregnant woman is concerned, this is an active phase for them. The woman's substantial participation matters as the force exerted to push the baby out determines this phase's extent.

The third stage: This involves the expulsion of the placenta from the uterus. I hope you are now familiar with the different stages of labor.

Reasons for the Failure of Normal Vaginal Delivery

1. Position of the baby—The labor slows down, or delivery fails if the baby is in breech or transverse position.
2. Size of the baby's head—The baby's large head or an abnormal angle of the presentation will slow down the labor process.
3. Your physical stature—An abnormal shape of your pelvis or a small size pelvis may not allow the baby to pass through the birth canal.

4. Your physical strength also determines the speed of labor. The stronger your abdominal muscles are, the better it will help to push the baby out.
5. Pain killers are believed to slow down the labor process since it hinders your ability to push the baby out.
6. Failure of the cervix to open up.
7. The environment of the labor room also influences the speed of delivery. A calmer and supportive environment and equally supportive people will help to hasten the labor process.

Labor, as you may assume, is not a highly complex process. With patience, relaxing techniques, and supportive people, you could make it very easy and comfortable A friend of mine mentioned a birth center in Delhi where the patients are placed in separate cubicles and are accompanied by their relatives.

Each cubicle is equipped with a music system and television, and they are allowed to watch television or listen to music during the contractions. She commented that the labor pain was not as excruciating as she had imagined because she was mentally relaxed during the whole process.

Such amenities should be made available in all the hospitals, helping to reduce the tensions associated with labor. Above all, the mental preparation of the patient matters a lot.

Now, in the next chapter, let us read about the C- section, which is usually taken up when the chances for a normal delivery become less or the baby is in some distress.

28

CAESAREAN SECTION

The term "Cesarean section" or C-section might be familiar to you all. The term is named after Julius Caesar, as it is believed that he was the first one to be delivered via a C-section. Even though there are some debates on the period and the option of surgery available at that time, people prefer to associate C-sections with Julius Caesar. In reality, the term is taken from the Latin word "caedare", which means "to cut". As we all are aware, vaginal delivery is the natural method of delivery. However, a C-section is done by delivering a baby through a cut in the mother's abdomen. There are many cases where normal vaginal delivery is not the best option, and there are specific maternal indications to opt for a C-section delivery. The primary aim of a C-section is to deliver a healthy baby while also keeping the mother's health in mind.

A C-section is usually done when some complications are seen in the baby and/or the mother. However, I have encountered several women who prefer to go for a C-section delivery as they are afraid of the pain accompanying a normal vaginal delivery. I recall meeting Eliza, who insisted on having a C-section delivery as she was not ready to bear the labor pain and contractions associated with a vaginal delivery. A team of Doctors, including me, tried to convince her about the positive aspects of normal delivery, as she had no other complications at that moment.

Some misconceptions about labor and pain were disturbing Eliza, and she was adamant about undergoing a C-section. We discussed the issue with her husband, who agreed to do things according to his wife's interest. Eliza's was not a unique case. I have seen many such women in the last 10 years. In 1985, the World Health Organization (WHO) stated:

"There is no justification for any region to have CS rates higher than 10-15%."
[World Health Organization. Appropriate technology for birth. Lancet 1985; 2 (8452): 436-7].

I have seen many couples opting for a C-section so that their baby will be born on auspicious days like Navaratri, New year, Christmas, etc. I remember Rahul and Riya, a couple from Delhi, who visited me at my clinic. Rahul was my cousin's friend, and hence, was also a close acquaintance of mine. Both of them were IT professionals and had been living in Bangalore. They came to meet me when Riya was eight months pregnant. Rahul asked about the possibilities of a C-section delivery as they were nearing the due date. I informed them of the positive side of going for a normal delivery rather than opting for a C-section.

Later Rahul mentioned that during their wedding, an astrologer had predicted that if their first baby was born during Navratri, they would inherit the ancestral property. So, when they started planning the pregnancy, they kept this prediction in mind. Everything went well; however, there was a slight miscalculation regarding the dates. Now, Riya's due date was five weeks after Navratri. Hence, they started thinking about a C-section so that the baby would be born during Navratri itself.

I informed them about the complications of getting the baby out five weeks before the estimated due date. Your child's health and safety should be the priority; hence, never give undue importance to the astrologers' predictions by tampering with the child's health.

A question that I usually encounter from the pregnant couple who come for their last pregnancy scan is, "Is it going to be a normal delivery?" Remember that a scanning Doctor is not the one who decides the type of delivery you will have. Even if the last scan shows an 80 percent chance for vaginal delivery, it can change depending on the health of the mother and the baby.

The chances for a vaginal delivery are more than 80 percent in the following conditions:

a. If it is your first pregnancy
b. If the baby head is positioned down (cephalic presentation)
c. If the pregnancy has crossed 37 weeks (full-term)
d. If the labor pain starts on its own

Likewise, several factors indicate a C-section delivery. Some among them are mentioned here:

1. The baby's head is unfavorable for vaginal delivery, making it difficult to pass through the birth canal.
2. Breech or foot presentation of the baby: These babies are usually born by C- section. Sometimes your Doctor can turn the baby by putting pressure on your tummy. This maneuver is called the external cephalic version (ECV). If the baby fails to turn, then a C- section is considered.
3. When there is a slow progress of labor or when the labor stops.
4. Abnormal heart response of the baby in the non-stress test (NST).
5. When you are carrying multiple pregnancies.
6. When there is a severe health problem in the mother like uncontrolled Diabetes mellitus, hypertension, heart or lung diseases, etc.
7. In case of placenta previa or abruption of the placenta.
8. Umbilical cord problems: The cord may prolapse through the cervix or sometimes the cord loops around the baby, not allowing it to descend through the uterus.
9. Some babies are too large to come out of the vagina safely.
10. A previous C-section also warrants C-section delivery in subsequent pregnancies.

In short, a C-section surgery is conducted if there are risk factors associated with the health of the mother or the baby. My wife had a C-section delivery as the cord was looped around the baby's neck. She had a prolonged first stage of labor which indicated a sign of distress for the baby. When I performed an ultrasound scan during this time, I happened to find the loop around the baby's neck.

I informed her Obstetrician, who advised a C-section. We were expecting a vaginal delivery; however, we had to think of the next option due to the emergency. You might also experience such emergencies during labor, and hence, should be prepared for a C-section delivery if it is indicated.

Apart from emergencies, I have seen cases where women opt for C-section deliveries for various other reasons. This is called an elective C-section, where the time and date for undertaking the delivery are fixed earlier. One of the primary reasons is that women want to avoid labor pain. I remember meeting Achu, who visited the hospital thrice during her ninth month complaining about pain. She had Braxton-Hicks pain; however, her Obstetrician realized that she had terrible fear about the labor.

The Doctor also feared that the panic of the mother might create distress in the baby. Hence, after consulting with her family members, they decided to conduct a C-section delivery. I have seen many patients like Achu while working in the hospital. When fear is the primary reason, delivering the baby on an auspicious day becomes another reason for an elective C-section.

Even though C-section is a safe procedure, it has some risk factors associated with it. Even normal vaginal delivery has certain risk factors associated with it. Some of the significant risks of a C-section delivery are listed here:

a) Surgery-related injury to the urinary bladder or intestine loops
b) Wound infection of the C-section scar
c) Delayed wound healing
d) Pain at the surgical site
e) Excess blood loss.
f) Blood clots in the calf veins
g) Infection of the endometrial lining (endometritis)
h) Incomplete removal of the placenta due to adhesions, resulting in removal of the uterus.

Just like the mother, the baby also faces some risks in a C-section delivery such as cut and scratch injuries and temporary breathing problems.

Let us quickly go through the different procedures that happen before, during, and after a C-section.

DUE DATE

1. **Preparation for surgery:** The Anesthesiologist and your Doctor will discuss the type of anesthesia usually administered for surgeries like spinal, epidural, and general anesthesia. Spinal and epidural anesthesia are mostly preferred for C-sections. In such cases, the anesthesia will numb the body below the chest, but you are conscious and awake.

   An Obstetrician commented about meeting a patient Sumi, who asked whether she will be given an epidural during C-section. The reason she gave for wanting this type of anesthesia moved my friend. Sumi said, "My baby has been within me for the past nine months. Hence, before my relatives and friends see it, I want to see my baby when I am fully conscious." General anesthesia is usually preferred during an emergency C-section, where you will be completely unconscious.
2. As part of the preparation, an intravenous line will be inserted into your hand. A blood sample is taken for lab tests, mainly to check for any prevailing infections. You will be administered relevant medicines to prevent complications, and your vitals, such as pulse, blood pressure, and ECG, are monitored. A urinary catheter is also inserted into your bladder, as you will not be able to move for nearly 24 hours after the C-section.
3. The complete C-section procedure may take 30 to 45 minutes, depending on your surgeon and the surgical team's skill and efficiency. However, your baby is delivered within 10 minutes of the start of the procedure. If you are awake during surgery, you will be able to hold your baby after the baby's primary resuscitation.
4. The typical hospital stay after surgery is two to three days, the duration of which depends on your health. It is essential to take good care of yourself to recover soon. Pain at the surgical site is the most common symptom after the anesthesia effect wears off. You will be given pain medication to make you feel comfortable.
5. There will be a slight vaginal discharge called lochia—a brownish red or clear discharge. It is normal to have a slight discharge for a few days to a few weeks after a C-section.
6. The bandage on the incision is removed within a day or two

after surgery. Your Doctor will assess the wound healing. You may feel a slight itching sensation, which is normal.

However, do not scratch the wound as it may get infected. The application of lotion will relieve the symptoms and help the wound heal faster. Some discomfort at the surgery site will persist for a few weeks after surgery. Just like with any other surgery, there are certain things you should do and some that you should avoid during the healing process.

1. A brief period of walking is encouraged after surgery to help recover your lung function and digestive function. It will help promote early wound healing and regain urinary bladder function.
2. Eating healthy will help you recover sooner.
3. Avoid lifting heavy objects and physical straining. Avoid physical exercise till your Doctor gives permission.
4. Take medicines as prescribed by the Doctor.
5. Avoid sex for three months.
6. Do not drive for one-to-two weeks after surgery.

However, you may experience some symptoms like painful urination, severe vaginal discharge, fever of more than 100° Fahrenheit, discharge from the incision site, and severe pain in the abdomen. In that case, you should immediately report these matters to your Doctor. C-section should not be a hurdle to enjoy the good moments with your new baby—it is only a medium for more happiness.

Now that you are familiar with labor, delivery, and C-sections, let us move to another major topic worth mentioning: Cord-Blood Sampling. Let us analyze the importance of this procedure in the next chapter.

29

CORD-BLOOD SAMPLING

You might have heard your friend or colleague talking about stem-cell banking. You might have received a call from the hospital about stem-cell banking for your baby. Many pregnant women during their third trimester ask for an opinion about stem-cell banking and whether they should opt for it. I remember Harsha, a patient of mine, asking me about stem-cell banking.

We had a brief conversation about this topic. I realized that Harsha had done good research on stem-cell banking, and I acknowledged her knowledge of that. She thanked 'Google Doctor' for offering her ample knowledge about this topic. Let me share my views on stem-cell banking. Stem-cell banking is the process of collecting the umbilical cord blood at the time of delivery and preserving the stem cells and other cells for future medical use.

The stem cells from the cord blood are called precursor cells, and they produce muscle cells, blood cells, bone cells, and so on. It has been scientifically proven that stored cells have the potential to cure many life-threatening diseases.

Many hospitals in developed countries like the United States of America and the United Kingdom have collected the newborn's stem cells for quite a long time. Hence, whenever the baby encounters life-threatening medical issues, the Doctors use stem cells to treat disease conditions.

Currently, stem cells are mostly used for the treatment of blood-related diseases like thalassemia and leukemia. Although private laboratories claim that stem-cell banking is used to cure hundreds of disorders, the truth is that they all are still in the experimental stage.

Stem cells can be stored in private labs or not-for-profit public cord-blood banks. You should remember that the cord blood of your baby will not be transplanted to cure your baby's disease. So, community stem-cell banking exists, which is similar to blood banks. Here, the stem cells from different donors are used to treat the condition.

Our government encourages parents to donate cord blood to public cord-blood banks for non-commercial purposes. Donating cord blood to public banks is free. Most stem-cell transplantation is done for unrelated donors from community cord-blood banks. There are very few instances where transplantation is done using the same baby's cells. So do not be misled by the idea that preserving your baby's stem cells will help cure the health conditions of your baby. Donating your baby's cord blood to the public bank is a noble cause to save another child's life.

Of course, your baby could also reap the benefit from a public bank in the future. Another important concept that should be learned with regard to the post-delivery phase is how to take care of the newborn. Sufficient knowledge is required about this process. Hence, in the next chapter, let us discuss how you could take care of the newborn and the different obstacles you might encounter while providing a healthy living condition to your baby.

PART 5

30

NEWBORN CARE

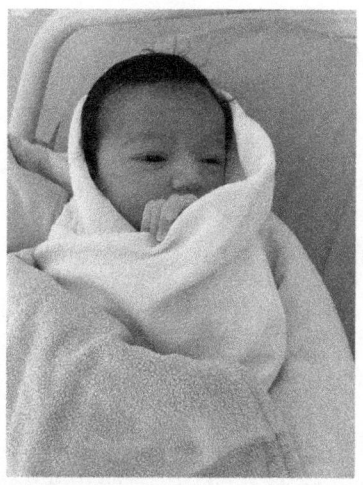

The neonatal period is characterized by the transition to an extrauterine environment and adjustment with the outside world. It is a critical period with significant risks for the newborn, and the care given during this time has a long-term effect on the physical and mental development of the baby. The term 'Neonate' refers to babies who belong to the age group from birth to one month old. It is a time that arrives after the long wait, and finally, your baby is in your arms.

You might be surprised to find your baby has wrinkled skin, puffy eyes, stubby nose, and a boat-shaped head. There is no need to be disappointed; your baby will become beautiful and more attractive as the weeks progress. I remember the daughter of Padma, who was born after prolonged labor. The baby did not breathe for a while after birth. Padma's husband, Kaushik, was a close acquaintance of mine, and he informed me. I called the concerned Pediatrician, who told me about the long delivery time to get the baby out. However, after ten minutes, the baby started breathing. The credit should go to the neonatal specialist and his team. The usual newborn care procedures include cutting the umbilical cord, which is then immediately clamped. After clamping, it is crucial to keep the clamped cord dry. Vitamin K injection is given to all newborn babies to boost their blood clotting mechanism. After these procedures, the baby will be moved to the nursery. An identity band mentioning the baby's gender, the baby's birth weight, and the mother's name will be put around the baby's leg.

Newborn Screening Tests

Your baby is tested for various metabolic disorders. These are called newborn screening tests. There are at least 50–60 tests that the baby will undergo within the first 48 hours, while you stay in the hospital. The number of tests done depends on hospital protocol. These tests are done to ensure that your baby doesn't have any life-threatening metabolic disorders. A single sample of blood is enough to test all these conditions. Your baby will also be screened for impaired hearing and congenital heart disease.

The first consultation with your Pediatrician will be scheduled within one week of your discharge from the hospital. It is normal for your baby to lose 5%–10% of its birthweight while in the hospital. It will take one to two weeks to regain the weight and thrive normally. Your baby will be checked for jaundice, a common but often temporary condition where your baby's skin appears yellow. A blood test to check bilirubin levels will help in knowing the severity of jaundice. Your baby should be able to move its arms and legs symmetrically. Parents often wonder whether their babies can see and respond to objects and gestures. The fact is that newborns primarily have a central vision and can see things within a distance of 8 to 15 inches.

The newborn babies can lift their heads momentarily while lying on their tummy. These physical characteristics are known as developmental milestones, and observing the milestones ensures good neuromuscular development.

The developmental milestones follow more or less the same pattern for most babies. However, the pace may slightly differ. If there is a delay in achieving these milestones, your Doctor will consider further evaluations to identify the problem. Hence periodic visits to the Doctor are needed, which might sometimes be accompanied by different tests. Your baby doesn't do much in the first few weeks except for eating, sleeping, pooping, and peeing. You will find your newborn sleeping for around 16–18 hours in a day; this sleep is essential for the development of the baby's brain.

Although babies don't seem to understand the language, make it a point to speak to your baby and enjoy motherhood. Make sure to feed your baby every two to three hours.

Thumb-sucking: It is natural for your baby to suck the thumb. They are born with the natural reflex of sucking. It acts as a pacifier. It is a sign for you to feed the baby.

Caring for the Baby in the Initial Few Hours of Life

After the initial stabilization procedures, the baby will be examined from head to toe, and all the findings will be recorded in the neonatal sheet. If all the results appear normal, the baby will then be shifted to its mother's side. However, the shifting time depends on the type of delivery and the baby's health. There are certain cases where the babies require special support; hence, they will be kept in the neonatal ICU until the neonatal specialist approves to shift the baby. Those babies born prematurely will be kept in the nursery or incubator until their development is complete.

Babies who are moved to the mother's side will be breastfed as early as possible to strengthen the bond between them. There are cases where mothers will not be able to feed the baby initially. Even though this is the case, never stop trying; only continuous feeding efforts will enhance continuous milk flow. I recall meeting Aabha, a new mother, who seemed to be disturbed in the post-operative recovery room. She had a C-section and was kept in the post-operative room for further monitoring.

When the baby was first given for breastfeeding in the post-operative room, she could not feed her baby, and she started worrying about how her baby would survive without her milk.

I was attending to a patient there and came to know about her from the nurses. I met her and talked to her. Many women have the same fear. Usually, the baby is kept close to the mother in the initial few hours. My wife once commented about her ecstasy when she held our daughter for the first time in her hands. Soon after the delivery, the parents will be informed about the importance of cord care, exclusive breastfeeding, intervals to be kept between consequent feeding, feeding positions to be used or avoided, the importance of burping, benefits and timing of oil massaging before discharge, etc.

It is essential to follow these recommendations as they are crucial to the well-being of the baby and the mother. A new baby will only be discharged from the hospital if proper feeding is established. According to the feeding pattern, the baby has to urinate six to eight times a day and follow a good sleeping pattern. Before discharge, the baby receives the vaccines that are given at birth. Physiological assessment of jaundice and bilirubin monitoring is also done before leaving the hospital. Newborn babies with no significant jaundice or other illnesses are usually discharged on the third day after birth. Some of the follow-up pieces of advice given to parents include

a) Feeding every two hours
b) Keeping the baby warm
c) Taking care of the baby's skin
d) Taking proper follow-up for jaundice check-ups
e) Expect weight loss for a week
f) Periodicity, consistency, and quantity of passing stool and urine might vary
g) Care of the cord
h) Explanation of danger signs

Newborn Issues: I would like to mention some of the common problems newborns could face during the initial days after their birth.

Neonatal Jaundice

Jaundice is a condition that occurs when the bilirubin is accumulated in a higher amount. In most cases, neonatal jaundice appears to be very mild. The bilirubin level is checked through a blood sample. A milder form of jaundice will settle on its own. The severe form of jaundice is treated through phototherapy. Likewise, the Doctors will also advise you to feed the baby frequently to help pass the excess bilirubin through stools. In case of uncontrolled severe jaundice, the Doctor will recommend an exchange blood transfusion to lower the bilirubin count.

A newborn baby is prone to several types of infections as its immune system is not adequately developed. Just like an adult, any kind of infection is harmful to a newborn baby. Always be on guard for symptoms of diseases, which should be treated with proper medications and antibiotics. Sometimes the infants have to be admitted to the hospitals for further treatment and procedures. As a mother, there are many things you can do while your baby is hospitalized.

1. Spend enough time with your baby by touching and talking to them. Skin-to-skin contact has a significant effect on improving the health condition of your baby.
2. Talk to your Neonatal Specialist or Pediatrician to know more about the baby's health condition.

Respiratory Distress Syndrome

This is one of the common medical conditions in premature babies. Premature infants with immature lungs lack surfactant, a lung enzyme that provides elasticity to the lungs and aids in easy breathing. Respiratory distress syndrome is usually managed with oxygen supplementation. Severe cases need ventilator/respirator support.

Intracranial Hemorrhage

Premature babies are at risk of developing bleeding in their brains. Whatever the severity of intracranial bleeding, the Doctors will observe it and advise follow-up scans to check the condition's progress.

Sometimes, large intracranial bleeds can result in cerebral palsy, spasticity, and intellectual disability.

Retinopathy of Prematurity

This medical condition refers to the abnormal growth of blood vessels in a baby's eyes. It has been medically proven that babies born between the gestation age of 23 to 26 weeks are prone to develop retinopathy of prematurity. All preterm babies are screened for retinopathy of prematurity by an Ophthalmologist.

IMMUNIZATION CHART FOR BABIES- BASED ON THE GUIDELINES PROVIDED BY THE INDIAN ACADEMY OF PEDIATRICS

Age Recommended	Vaccine	Age Recommended	Vaccine
Birth	BCG	9 months	Measles
Birth	Hepatitis B_1	9 months	OPV
Birth	OPV	12-18 months	Hepatitis A_1
6 weeks	Hepatitis B_2	15 months	$Varicella_1$
6 weeks	HiB_1	15 months	MMR 1st dose
6 weeks	DPT_1/ $DTAP_1$	18 months	IPV/ OPV
6 weeks	IPV	18 months	DPT_{B1}/ $DTaP_{B1}$

DUE DATE

	Vaccine	Age	Vaccine
	Rotavirus$_1$	12-18 months	HiB$_B$
	Pneumococcal$_1$		Pneumococcal$_B$
10 weeks	IPV	12–24 months	Typhoid$_1$
	DPT$_2$/ DTaP$_2$		Hepatitis A$_2$
	HiB$_2$	2 years	Meningococcal Conjugate vaccine ACWY
	Rotavirus$_2$	4–6 years	MMR 2nd dose
	Pneumococcal$_2$		Varicella$_2$
14 weeks	IPV	5 years	IPV/OPV
	DPT$_3$/ DTaP$_3$		DPT$_{B2}$/ DTaP$_{B2}$
	HIB$_3$		Typhoid$_2$
	Rotavirus$_3$	8 years	Typhoid$_3$
	Pneumococcal$_3$	10 years and above (Girls)	HPV$_1$ HPV$_2$ HPV$_3$

6 months	Hepatitis B$_3$	10 years	TdaP
	IPV/OPV	11 years	Typhoid$_4$
	Influenza$_1$	14 years	Typhoid$_5$
7 months	Influenza$_2$	16 years	TdaP

Worrisome Signs and Symptoms Indicating your Baby is Sick and Needs Medical Attention

1. Irritable with excessive crying that cannot be comforted
2. Not playful as usual
3. Abnormally dull and inactive
4. Unusual breathing sound
5. Unusually hot or cold skin
6. Persistent vomiting or loose stools
7. Refusing feeds

Standard Frequency of Pediatric Consultation

These consultations are meant to evaluate the baby's growth and development (milestones) and ensure vaccinations as per schedule.

1. First consultation: Within 10 days from the day of birth
2. Second consultation: Between 8 weeks and 10 weeks
3. Third consultation: Between 10 weeks and 12 weeks
4. Fourth consultation: Between 3 and 4 months
5. Fifth consultation: Between 8 and 9 months
6. Sixth consultation: Between 12 and 15 months
7. Seventh consultation: At 18 months
8. Eighth consultation: At 2 years.

However, if your baby is unwell or manifests worrisome signs and symptoms, it should be immediately reported to the Doctor.

There are many more complications that are associated with premature birth. Newborn care is of utmost importance as it determines the health of the baby throughout its life. In the next chapter, let us learn about the different birth control methods that could be used after the delivery.

31

BIRTH CONTROL AFTER DELIVERY

My grandparents had eight babies who were born one year apart. I always wondered how she managed to look after all these kids together. Out of curiosity, I inquired her of the same. She smiled and said that birth control measures were not available during their time, so it happened independently. When she realized she was pregnant, she was ready to invite the new baby to their family. She mentioned that it was her mental preparedness that mattered. I was so happy to hear this answer.

However, this led me to request my colleague Dr. Puja Rathi, an Obstetrician, to share her knowledge about birth control measures practiced after pregnancy.

Many communities restrict the couple's sexual relations for the first three months following the pregnancy. I had a colleague who invited me for a function at his home. I do not recall the function's name; however, he mentioned that it was arranged for his baby's arrival at his house after three months of his birth. As I was not aware of such events, I asked him for more details. According to the rituals in his community, the wife would go to her house while she was seven months pregnant. She could only return after three months post-delivery.

The ancestors, who realized the need to provide rest to the women, introduced this custom. Accordingly, the new mother would get ample time to get attached to the newborn and enough rest for the injuries caused by the delivery to heal. The function, which happens once she returns home, is also a sign of re-establishing the sexual life of the couple.

Many communities and religions have the same approach to postpartum sexual life to restrict another pregnancy soon after the first one. In fact, Doctors advise abstinence from sex till three months after the birth of the baby.

There is a common belief that breastfeeding mothers will not get pregnant in the first six months as ovulation is suppressed during this phase. This claim is not the absolute truth because I have witnessed many women getting pregnant within the first six months of postpartum.

I recall meeting Amritha, who came to me for her early pregnancy scan. She was gloomy throughout the procedure, and I asked her about the cause for her distressed condition. I found it very difficult to converse with her as her words were not clear due to the sobbing which accompanied it. When I talked with her husband, I realized that she had a six-month-old baby, and the current pregnancy was an accidental event.

I kept thinking about her for the next few days. When my wife found me lost in thought, she inquired about the cause. When I revealed the incident, she lectured me about getting so emotional, especially when I had to be a pillar of support for my patients. Nevertheless, this incident led me to think more about such issues faced by women in the postpartum period. That is why I thought of educating my readers by requesting my colleague to contribute a chapter.

If you are a breastfeeding mother, you can adopt contraceptive techniques such as condoms, diaphragms, contraceptive injections, intrauterine devices, permanent sterilization, etc. It would help if you talked to your Obstetrician about the different methods available, how they work, which method is suitable for you, how soon you can start using the contraceptive method, possible side effects, etc. The more you learn about the various contraceptive methods, the better prepared you will be to choose what is best for you.

Among non-breastfeeding women, ovulation occurs as early as six weeks after delivery. However, it depends from person to person.

An Obstetrician must provide an insight into the time gap needed for the subsequent pregnancy, which varies from woman to woman.

The Obstetrician should be aware of the couple's social, sexual, and familial history before prescribing a contraceptive method.

Most of these methods are prescribed after knowing about the patient's health conditions, age, type of delivery, previous pregnancy issues, etc. Remember that no contraceptive method is 100 percent successful or safe. The following are the different types of birth-control methods:

> **Abstinence:**
>> **Abstinence** is the simplest and the safest form of birth control where the couple completely refrain from sexual intercourse. Another method that many couples practice to avoid pregnancy is self-enforced restrainment from ejaculating semen into the vaginal canal to prevent pregnancy. This is a very unreliable method of controlling pregnancy.

> **Barrier Method:**
>> Another method you could adopt is the **barrier method**. Men and women can use this contraceptive method which protects them against pregnancy and sexually transmitted diseases. Women use the diaphragm, and cervical cap, as a mode of barrier method. It is recommended to adopt this method only six to eight weeks after the delivery. This method of contraception prevents sperm from entering the uterus. Female condoms, sponges, spermicidal foam, male condoms, etc., are also part of this contraception method. This method has been shown to have 98 percent success in preventing pregnancy.

> **Lactational Amenorrhea:**
>> The next method is the **lactational amenorrhea** method, which is very controversial concerning its success rate. Here, breastfeeding is considered a contraceptive method. This method is beneficial only if you entirely breastfeed your baby and your periods have not resumed up to six months. Even though periods do not resume, ovulation might happen.

So, I would suggest that you not rely on this contraceptive method and select other methods to prevent pregnancy.

- **Pills and Injections:**
  Pills and injections are hormonal methods of birth control. Three different techniques are used in this method.
  a) **Combined Oral Contraceptive Pills:**
     This can be used one month after delivery in a non-breastfeeding woman. The efficacy rate of this method is 99 percent. However, there is not enough clinical evidence about the impact of combined pills on breastfeeding mothers, as it might harm the quantity and quality of breast milk. Hence, it is essential that the couple make an unanimous decision regarding combined contraceptive pills after weighing all the pros and cons.

  b) **Progesterone-Only Pills:**
     The second hormonal method you could adopt is the progesterone-only pill; its effectiveness is supposed to be 99 percent. The new mother could start using this pill any time after the delivery.

  c) **Depot Medroxyprogesterone (DMPA):**
     This injection is administered soon after a baby's birth in a non-breastfeeding woman. A breastfeeding woman should adopt this method only after six weeks of delivery.

- **Intra-Uterine Devices (IUDs):**
  These are small mechanical devices inserted into the uterine cavity. These include
  a) **Copper-containing devices commonly called Cu-T**
  b) **Hormone releasing IUDs**

  These can be inserted four weeks after the delivery. If the device is inserted before this phase, it can result in its expulsion or perforation of the uterus.

- **Female Sterilization:**
  It is a permanent surgical procedure for birth control. The approach mentioned here is termed tubectomy.

In this process, the fallopian tubes are blocked, which prevents the egg from reaching the uterus. The decision rests with the couple whether to go forward with this method or not. This process is irreversible, and the failure rate and the complications associated with the surgical procedure are minimal.

If you are having a C-section delivery, tubectomy is usually performed at the same time. However, prior counseling is needed, and your Obstetrician will suggest you undergo this counseling at least two weeks before the procedure.

For women with normal vaginal delivery, another process termed mini-laparotomy is conducted, where the procedure is carried out with a small incision over the abdomen. It is scientifically proven that the lifetime failure of this method is one in two hundred. The tubectomy is also beneficial in protecting women against ovarian tumors and pelvic infections.

Another fact associated with tubectomy is that this method does not affect your menstrual cycle, unlike hormonal contraceptive methods. I hope you have a good understanding of the different birth control methods and their uses.

If you are not planning a new pregnancy soon after the delivery, better be on guard. In the next chapter, I will discuss another important concept that comes after delivery, breastfeeding.

32

BREASTFEEDING

Breastfeeding is often termed the "miracle of nature" that nourishes the newborn baby. I remember meeting Sushama, who was upset during her ninth-month scan. I enquired about the issue and realized that she was doubtful whether the baby would suck the milk from her breast.

I tried to convey that sucking is an automatic function, which does not require any training. Many pregnant women have asked me the same question regarding breastfeeding. Some mothers could not produce enough milk, and these doubts and tensions will only reduce milk production.

Breast milk alone provides all the nutrients a baby needs for the first six months, and it protects against a range of illnesses. Research suggests that breastfed babies have better mental development than that in non-breastfed babies. Bottle feeding often results in babyhood obesity. One of my professors mentioned a case where the grandparents decided to feed the baby with cow's milk soon after the delivery.

They believed that cow's milk would be more nutritious than mother's milk. This claim, however, is not true as cow's milk might be beneficial for the newborn calf and not for the human baby. Colostrum, the first milk produced by the mother, contains antibodies that help protect the baby from infections.

No other type of milk could substitute the mother's milk as it is nutritious and needed. It is recommended to breastfeed your baby for the first six months exclusively. If you could continue breastfeeding your baby even after six months, it would be an added advantage.

Soon after the delivery, the baby will be kept closer to you so that you can develop a good emotional bond with your baby. Remember that latching is the best way to feed your baby where the baby takes the nipple, including the entire areola, for sucking.

Some Doctors suggest not to feed the baby before it cries for it. This dictum is not right in all circumstances. You need not wait for the baby to cry for the feed. Your baby will start showing certain signs that it is hungry, apart from the crying.

There are signs of understanding that your baby is hungry. The baby tries to suck its finger or anything that is kept near the mouth. This phenomenon is called the suckling reflex. When the baby becomes hungry, it mistakes its finger or a nearby object for the nipple.

Your baby starts keeping the tongue out or turning its head repeatedly. If you see these actions, you should breastfeed immediately. Crying is often the last sign the baby shows when it is hungry. Doctors always suggest feeding the baby once every two hours. While feeding, make sure to feed through both breasts, alternately. If only one breast is continuously used for feeding, you might feel pain in the unused breast due to excessive congestion of milk.

Feeding the baby is a tiresome task, and hence, the mother should find a comfortable position to do the same. Make yourself comfortable while breastfeeding. Lie down on your side while the baby is facing you. Most Doctors advise mothers to sit and breastfeed. Sit in a comfortable position while supporting the baby's head on your arms. You can use soft pillows to support your back and arms. A mother's comfort and relaxed mood positively affect milk production. Below are some steps that you could follow while breastfeeding.

Pat your breasts with a soft cloth after every feed to prevent skin cracking. Drink water after every feed to keep yourself hydrated.

Once you are admitted to the hospital, soon after the delivery, you could ask for help from a nurse or a lactation counselor on feeding techniques. If your baby passes urine at least six times a day, it is indicative of receiving adequate feeds.

If there is any difficulty in expressing the milk, a manual or automatic breast pump could be used to express the milk from the breast. I hope now you are acquainted with the different things to be noted when you start your newborn care. In the next part, let us analyze some common issues in pregnancy. We will, first, discuss multiple pregnancies in the next chapter.

33

MULTIPLE PREGNANCY

Pregnancy is blissful, and the news of a multiple pregnancy calls for mixed emotions from the parents' side. There are certain misconceptions and myths about multiple pregnancies. One of my relatives used to consume twin bananas to get pregnant with twins. However, it has been deemed a myth as it does not have any scientific backing. The term multiple pregnancy is not concerned with twin babies alone. It basically means that the pregnant woman is carrying more than one baby in her womb—twins, triplets, quadruplets, or more.

Recently, I read about a woman who gave birth to four babies at a time. Hence, when you hear the phrase multiple pregnancy, please do not mistake it for twin babies alone. It is observed that women who conceive after the IVF treatment are more often found to have multiple pregnancies. The most common type of multiple pregnancy is a twin pregnancy.

Twin pregnancies can be of two types: identical twins and non-identical twins. Surveys have clearly stated that the chances of having non-identical twins are higher compared to that of having identical twins. In India, the incidence of birthing identical twins and non-identical twins is 4 in 1000 and 9 in 1000 births, respectively. Twin pregnancies happen in two different ways, and this denotes whether the babies are identical or non-identical.

Identical twin pregnancy occurs when the single egg gets fertilized by a single sperm and eventually splits to form two zygotes. Babies born in such an event will have similar genetic composition and physical characteristics. There are cases when identical twins fail to separate, resulting in conjoined twins or Siamese twins.

However, the instances of conjoined twins are very rare. Non-identical twins are formed when two different eggs get fertilized by two different sperms simultaneously. Usually, during a menstrual cycle, the female body will produce only one egg. In some exceptional cases, the ovaries release two or more eggs simultaneously, which get fertilized together when the sperms enter the body.

The resulting pregnancy from such an exceptional fertilization process results in non-identical twins. Many parents are unaware of this phenomenon, and hence, when they hear the term twins, they believe that the babies will look alike. Unlike the pregnancy myth, certain groups of people have more chances of developing multiple pregnancies. For instance, if there are cases of multiple pregnancies in your family or your husband's family, you have more chances of having a multiple pregnancy. Likewise, if you or your partner are one among twins or triplets, the chances of you having have a multiple pregnancy are high. Elderly mothers, who are more than 35 years of age, can also conceive multiple pregnancies.

As mentioned earlier, many women, who have conceived through IVF treatment, are also found to have multiple pregnancies. Multiple pregnancies are often diagnosed through ultrasonography. The ultrasound scan helps to understand the growth and well-being of the babies inside the womb. Multiple pregnancies are often diagnosed as early as the fifth week when multiple pregnancy sacs are identified within the uterus. However, Doctors usually wait till the eighth week to confirm.

In a multiple pregnancy, the babies often carry slightly higher risks of developing congenital disabilities than the babies in singleton pregnancies do.

An ultrasound scan helps to detect any abnormalities early in the pregnancy. The ultrasound scan also helps analyze the growth and development of the multiple babies present in the womb. I had a patient who carried triplets in her womb. Her Obstetrician wanted her to undertake an ultrasound scan every month to evaluate the growth and development of the babies.

Along with all these factors, an ultrasound scan helps understand the head positions when these pregnancies approach their due date.

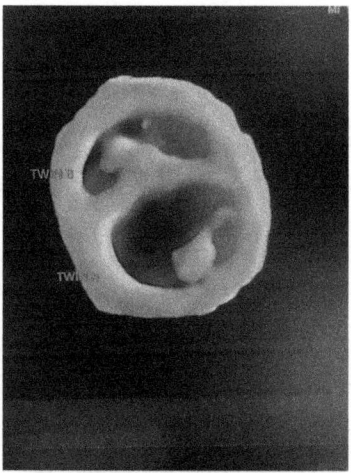

3-D early pregnancy scan showing Twin Gestation

The pregnancy signs and symptoms are often exaggerated in multiple pregnancies, as compared to a singleton pregnancy. The pregnant woman will experience severe bodily discomforts with the growth of the babies inside her womb. Unlike a normal pregnancy, women who conceive multiple babies are often called to visit the Doctor more frequently. As mentioned earlier, ultrasound scans are also undertaken more frequently as fetal growth restriction is common in multiple pregnancies. Sometimes, only one baby among the multiple babies will have growth restrictions. In such cases, Doctors often think of treatment and surgical procedures.

The growing babies require more nutrition and energy to finish up the last-minute requirements they need for their entry into the world. Hence, women with multiple pregnancies will experience severe tiredness compared to that in women with a singleton pregnancy. The nutrition demand will be higher for women who have multiple babies in their wombs. Eating right is the best way to meet this demand. Make sure not to mistake eating right with eating more. Only eating right will enable you to maintain the needed weight and ensure that your babies get enough nutrition for their growth and development. Eating more will only lead to untoward weight gain, which results in pregnancy complications.

One of the crucial questions often asked by pregnant women carrying multiple babies is, "Will there be any problem with my pregnancy?" I remember meeting Neha, who was found to have two babies in her womb. In her first scan, I disclosed the news to her and her husband.

I could see happiness in her husband Ratan's face; however, Neha seemed tense and gloomy. Out of curiosity, I asked her about the gloomy mood. She replied that she was worried and anxious about her twin pregnancy. Many issues often accompany multiple pregnancies. With proper care and treatment methods, most of the issues can be overcome. One of the significant issues associated with multiple pregnancies is preterm delivery. As there is more than one baby in the uterus, the cervix cannot withhold the weight, and there is a chance that the cervix might open up early in the pregnancy. Hence, when a woman is diagnosed with a multiple pregnancy, many Doctors suggest putting a cervical suture to avoid premature birth. Another issue that can be associated with multiple pregnancies is the early onset of labor.

There has been much research to show that pregnant women carrying multiple babies might experience early labor compared to women with singleton pregnancies. The chances of developing gestational Diabetes and hypertension will also be higher. Losing a baby during pregnancy might be a traumatic experience for the mother. Hence, proper care should be undertaken for pregnant women, especially those carrying multiple babies. The Obstetrician decides the type of delivery to be undertaken for during multiple pregnancies. It solely depends on the position, weight, and well-being of the babies within the uterus. Vaginal delivery is possible if the first baby's head is closest to the birth canal. Once the first baby is born, the other twin will come out effortlessly.

Make sure that you get enough sleep and rest. Make it a point to sleep when the babies are sleeping. Breastfeeding will be another issue you might experience. Usually, mothers having multiple babies will have more milk supply. However, if you experience reduced milk production, your Pediatrician might suggest milk supplements to ensure your babies' nutrient intake. Now let us discuss the topic of gestational diabetes in the next chapter.

34

GESTATIONAL DIABETES

Gestational Diabetes is a condition in which blood glucose levels are elevated during pregnancy—the carbohydrate metabolism changes during pregnancy to ensure a continuous supply of glucose to the baby.

As Indians, we are at a higher risk of developing Diabetes, especially, if there is a family history of Diabetes. Gestational Diabetes is a Type-2 Diabetes.

I recall meeting Dishita, who had gestational Diabetes from the fifth month of her pregnancy. She was only 23 years old, and she felt ashamed to inform her family members. When asked, she said, "How will I face my parents? My father became a Diabetic only in his early forties. How can I tell them that I am Diabetic at the age of 23?" It took me a good amount of time to explain about Diabetes in pregnancy.

After my counseling, Dishita seemed pensive. I continued my session and informed her that gestational Diabetes would mostly reverse once the baby was delivered.

I hoped that it was a comforting message to her, as she stopped her questions at that moment. I revealed that with a strong family history of Diabetes, gestational Diabetes is a common phenomenon. There are two types of Diabetes in pregnancy: Gestational Diabetes and Pre-Existing Diabetes.

1. **Gestational Diabetes** – This occurs only during pregnancy due to hormonal changes in the body. The condition is usually detected after 20—24 weeks of pregnancy. Most of the time, Diabetes reverses after the delivery of the baby.
2. **Pre-Existing Diabetes (pre-gestational)** – In this condition, the blood sugars are high even before pregnancy.

Here, the Diabetic condition is not a new phenomenon. The pregnant woman might have already been on medication or insulin injections. Always remember to mention these health conditions to your Doctor while going for a consultation. Above all, you should closely monitor your sugar levels to avoid the problems associated with uncontrolled Diabetes.

Normal Blood Sugar Levels in Pregnancy

BLOOD TEST	**NORMAL RANGE**
Fasting blood glucose level	90–110 mg/dL
Postprandial blood sugar	100–140 mg/dL

Any pregnant woman can develop Gestational Diabetes. However, the conditions that increase the risk of developing diabetes include the following:
 1. Overweight (high BMI)
 2. History of Diabetes in a previous pregnancy
 3. Family history of early-onset Diabetes
 4. Pre-existing high blood pressure & high cholesterol levels
 5. Women having PCOD
 6. Giving birth to a big baby (weight >4.0 kg)

A blood sugar test is done during your first visit to the Doctor. Checking blood sugar is a part of the routine check-up during your antenatal visits.

It is recommended to check blood sugar levels before becoming pregnant, especially if you have a family history of Diabetes, obesity, elevated cholesterol levels, or PCOD.

DUE DATE

Gestational Diabetic mothers usually carry a large baby, and there will be an increased amount of amniotic fluid (polyhydramnios). The insulin levels would be high in the baby of a Diabetic mother. This causes an increased glucose absorption by the body cells resulting in excessive growth of the baby, called macrosomia. The complications associated with uncontrolled Gestational Diabetes include

1. A shoulder injury to the baby during the vaginal delivery,
2. Polyhydramnios, or excess fluid around the baby,
3. Breathing difficulty in the baby as lung maturity is delayed,
4. Heart defects in the baby,
5. Increased risk of fetal death in the late trimester, etc.

It is essential to monitor blood glucose levels periodically. Fasting blood sugar (FBS) and postprandial blood sugar are the standard tests that help identify Diabetes. However, the Glucose Tolerance Test (GTT) is another gold standard for diagnosing Gestational Diabetes. The box added below gives a clear understanding of the GTT. FBS is often checked on an empty stomach in the morning. FBS value that is above 140 mg/dL is often considered Diabetic. Pregnant women are advised to maintain the value under 110 mg/dL so that the chances of developing gestational Diabetes will be lower.

ORAL GLUCOSE TOLERANCE TEST (OGTT)

The 75-gm glucose tolerance test
A fasting blood sugar test is conducted before the pregnant woman consumes 75 gm of glucose mixed with 150 mL of water. Two blood samples are collected in intervals of one hour after drinking the glucose water. A blood sugar level less than 140 mg/dL is considered normal. A blood sugar value between 140–190 mg/dL indicates the likelihood of developing gestational Diabetes, and a value above 190 mg/dL proves that you have diabetes.

The 50-gm glucose challenge test
In this test, fasting blood glucose level is not checked. The test can be done at any time of the day. The pregnant woman consumes 50 gm of glucose mixed with 150 mL of water. Blood sugar levels are checked after one hour. A blood sugar level below 140 mg/dL is considered normal. A value between 140 mg/dL and below 190 mg/dL suggests the need for a three-hour GTT to diagnose gestational diabetes. A value above 190 mg/dL confirms the diagnosis of gestational diabetes.

Home monitoring of blood sugar can be done using a Glucometer device. It is advisable to buy a glucometer. There is a misconception lurking around gestational Diabetes that it is difficult to manage. However, studies have pointed out that managing Diabetes during pregnancy is not an impossible task. Some facts you ought to know about managing Diabetes are mentioned below. It is important to follow these, especially during pregnancy.

1. Strict maintenance of blood sugar levels: The FBS should be less than 110 mg/dL, whereas the postprandial (after meal) blood sugar should be below 140 mg/dL.
2. A good diet. (Refer to the chapter "Eating Right During Pregnancy").
3. Regular Exercise (Refer to the chapter "Fitness during Pregnancy" and "Prenatal Yoga").
4. Drugs – Medicines are advised based on blood sugar levels. Insulin injection is preferred over oral medicines to manage gestational Diabetes.
5. It is also essential to get a heart check-up and eye check-up done as well.
6. Babies of diabetic mothers tend to put on weight very fast, creating preterm labor issues.

Even though the babies gain weight quickly, their organs are yet to be adequately developed. Hence, babies born in the second or early third trimester are often kept in the incubator until their organs function well. The health of these babies, when they are still in the womb, is monitored as follows:

- Regular ultrasound scans to check the baby's growth.
- Non-stress test (NST) is done regularly after 32 weeks of pregnancy.

Similar to gestational Diabetes, another major health issue often found in pregnancy is Hypertension. Like gestational Diabetes, if left untreated and unchecked, hypertension too creates havoc. Hence, let us think about this condition in the next chapter.

35

HYPERTENSION IN PREGNANCY

Hypertension is one of the common medical conditions in pregnancy. It can be defined as elevated blood pressure. Like diabetes, hypertension in pregnancy is of two types:

1. Pregnancy-Induced Hypertension (PIH)
2. Pre-existing Hypertension.

> **Normal Average Blood pressure:**
>
> Systolic BP - 100–140 mmHg
> Diastolic BP - 70–90 mmHg
> Gestational hypertension is diagnosed when the BP recording is 140/90 mmHg or more diagnosed after 20 weeks of pregnancy.

One of the primary questions that many Doctors encounter from pregnant women is, "Why did I develop hypertension?" There is no specific reason why hypertension happens. Some women complain about swelling in the legs, which they often self-diagnose as a symptom of hypertension.

PIH usually manifests after 24 weeks of pregnancy. Hypertension in pregnancy is often accompanied by specific signs and symptoms, which depend on the severity of the condition. In the olden days, especially when the medical field was not as advanced, hypertension in pregnancy went unnoticed. The milder form of PIH will present as ankle and foot swelling.

The moderate and severe forms can be found in pregnant women who complain about headaches, vision blurring, chest tightness, face swelling, etc. There will be excretion of proteins (albumin) in the urine in the moderate and severe forms of PIH. This leads to HELLP Syndrome, characterized by hemolysis, abnormal liver function, and low platelet counts.

Symptoms of severe cases of hypertension also include fits, vomiting, restlessness, etc. In rare cases, pregnant women may even fall unconscious due to very high blood pressure.

The impact of hypertension on the developing baby depends on the severity of hypertension. The baby will not have any complications with the milder form of hypertension. Severe hypertension causes fetus growth restriction resulting in an underweight baby.

The management of pre-existing hypertension and PIH is essentially the same. Let us look at some of the pointers associated with the treatment of hypertension in pregnancy.

1. Prevention is better than cure. It is an excellent practice to keep the blood pressure under control before becoming pregnant. Pre-existing hypertension complicates the outcome of pregnancy as compared to PIH. It is reassuring that in the majority of the cases, the pregnancy outcome will be good.
2. Every time you visit the Doctor, measuring the blood pressure (BP) is part of your check-up. So, you do not have to worry about the BP monitoring part. But make sure to visit your Doctor regularly as suggested.
3. Lifestyle management—Reduce weight and avoid a salty and spicy diet. Reduce oil-rich food.
4. Drugs—Anti-hypertensive drugs will help to control hypertension.
5. Buy a digital apparatus for self-monitoring of BP.
6. Monitor your fluid intake and urine output.

7. Get an abdomen ultrasound scan to check kidneys over time and ensure that nothing is missed. During your NT & NB scan, the sonologist records the Uterine artery Doppler, which predicts the risk of PIH. If there is a risk, you will be advised to take a low dose of aspirin (75 mg tablet) every day till the 36th week of pregnancy.

Low-dose aspirin acts as a blood thinner, reducing blood viscosity within the small vessels. It helps to lower blood pressure. The complications of hypertension are pre-eclampsia and seizures.

In uncontrolled hypertension, preterm delivery is advised to avoid the complications of eclampsia and pre-eclampsia. Fortunately, there is less risk of respiratory distress to the baby with gestational hypertension, and in fact, the lung matures early. Placental abruption is a rare complication experienced in complicated and severe cases of hypertension. This would result in stillbirth.

Another major obstacle that you may find during pregnancy is Fetus Growth Restriction. Let us discuss it in the next chapter.

36

FETUS GROWTH RESTRICTION (FGR)

You might have heard about Fetus Growth Restriction (FGR), where the baby does not grow to its full potential inside the uterus. A colleague of mine called me a couple of weeks ago to seek a second opinion about a case of FGR. I immediately reached the clinic to check the scan.

The woman was eight months pregnant; however, the baby's growth rate was meager from what was expected from an eight-month-old baby.

In the eighth month of gestation, the fetus is supposed to weigh 1.5 kg to 1.8 kg. Just like my colleague suspected, the baby's growth was retarded.

The couple understood the severity of the case from our discussion and became anxious. I often come across such pregnancies with fetal growth restrictions. One of the common questions these patients often ask me is whether they have done anything wrong leading to this particular situation regarding diet, medication, and lifestyle habits.

FGR cannot be completely prevented as it often happens for unknown reasons. Some pregnancies come under the high-risk category for developing FGR. They include

1. Mother having high blood pressure,
2. Poor nutrition of the mother,
3. Multiple pregnancies,
4. A mother who is suffering from long-standing diseases of the heart, liver, and kidney,
5. Placental and umbilical cord diseases resulting in poor blood circulation to the baby,
6. TORCH infections,
7. Chromosomal abnormalities in the fetus, etc.

Having mentioned all these factors, many a time, FGR has no underlying causes. There are a few signs and symptoms if you are carrying a growth-restricted fetus. Your Doctor will measure your tummy size (fundal height) at every prenatal visit, and it gives an idea of the fetus's growth.

If the mother is not gaining weight, there is suspicion of FGR. The definitive way to detect FGR is by undertaking ultrasonography. An ultrasound scan can help in knowing the baby's weight and quantifying the baby's blood flow.

Once FGR is diagnosed, the scanning Doctor will stage the severity of growth restriction depending on the baby's weight and Doppler changes. Based on the staging of the growth restriction, the baby will be monitored closely by an ultrasound scan. Depending on the gestational age, the baby is monitored frequently. Sometimes, your Doctor may ask you to get an ultrasound scan frequently until the baby is delivered.

If the ultrasound scan suggests that the baby is not in danger, the pregnancy may continue till 37 weeks. If the Doppler findings suggest otherwise, delivery is done by C-section to avoid complications like fetus death, respiratory distress, etc. Careful monitoring and early intervention may reduce the difficulties to the fetus.

Eliminating the risk factors and adopting a healthy lifestyle can reduce the occurrence of FGR. The good news is that the baby diagnosed with growth restriction will generally catch up with normal growth by two years of age. Understanding miscarriage is accompanied by coping with the same. Let us discuss this topic in the next chapter.

37

UNDERSTANDING MISCARRIAGE AND COPING WITH IT

Do you wonder why people use the term "carrying" as a synonym for pregnancy? But when put against the antonym of pregnancy, "carrying" is proper usage. The antonym of pregnancy, according to a thesaurus, also includes the term miscarriage. Losing a pregnancy is heartbreaking. It is an unfortunate incident that blows out the happiness of a family. On an average, about 1 in every 10 pregnancies ends in a miscarriage, meaning pregnancy loss is not a rare occurrence.

I recall meeting Zibiah, a mother-to-be, who came for her ultrasound scan in the fourth month due to excessive bleeding. She was aware that bleeding was not a good sign of pregnancy. So, she informed her Obstetrician when she noticed slight vaginal bleeding. However, by the time she reached the hospital, she was bleeding heavily. I was asked to conduct an ultrasound scan to know the condition, even though the parents-to-be and the Doctors were sure about the miscarriage. Soon after the scanning, I declared the news of miscarriage to the parents, and Zibiah immediately asked me if she had done something wrong.

She was doubtful about the food she consumed and the lifestyle habits she had been following. I was perplexed and revealed that miscarriages are unavoidable, and the actual cause behind them is not detectable all the time. The most common cause of pregnancy loss or miscarriage is chromosome abnormality, which hinders the normal growth of the fetus. Other factors that result in miscarriage include the following:

- Abnormal thyroid hormone levels
- Progesterone deficiency in mother
- Uncontrolled Diabetes mellitus
- Exposure to the hazards experienced in the environment and workplace, such as radiation or toxic agents
- Certain infections (e.g., TORCH infections)
- Uterus abnormalities
- Incompetent cervix
- Usage of certain medications
- Certain lifestyle habits also increase the risk of a miscarriage. Smoking puts nicotine and other chemicals into the bloodstream, causing the fetus to get less oxygen. This increases the chance of losing a pregnancy.
- Alcohol and illicit drug usage might also lead to miscarriages.

While miscarriages usually cannot be prevented, taking proper care of yourself and following your Doctor's instructions can reduce the risk of pregnancy loss. Many women would not even know they had a miscarriage because they assume the bleeding to be a normal menstrual flow. The common symptoms of miscarriage are abdomen cramps, spotting or heavier bleeding from the vagina, pelvic pain, weakness, or back pain. Many times, women become anxious about vaginal spotting.

Vaginal spotting need not always be a symptom of miscarriage since many women experience it during early pregnancy. If you experience any of these symptoms during your pregnancy, it is advisable to report the issue to your Doctor. Your Doctor will perform the pelvis examination, and an ultrasound scan will be conducted to confirm the miscarriage. Sometimes serum Beta-hCG blood tests may be required.

These tests give an accurate idea of whether the patient has undergone a miscarriage or not. Understanding miscarriage and getting the correct diagnosis are of great importance. Finding the exact cause for the miscarriage is not possible in some instances. However, it has been scientifically proven that the common cause for early pregnancy loss can be attributed to the unnatural genetic composition of the embryo, which hinders its growth.

You should be thankful for the miscarriage, as it is nature's way of stopping the growth of an abnormal pregnancy. Encountering a pregnancy loss is always followed by a period of grief. However, the duration of this period depends on many factors. Some among them are repeated miscarriages, losing a baby at the later trimester of pregnancy or during labor. It could also have a profound impact in case of a precious pregnancy like conceiving at an older age, getting pregnant after undertaking infertility treatment, etc.

In most circumstances, time becomes the healer, and as time passes, the depressive and sad moods associated with the pregnancy loss go away. Accepting the loss and believing that the best is yet to arrive is the maxim you should follow to overcome the depressive state of mind. The six stages of emotions associated with pregnancy loss are as listed:

1. **Denial:** When the news of pregnancy loss reaches you, you might be shocked. This condition leads to a denial of the fact that you have lost your baby. Most Obstetricians advise their patients to undergo a second scan to confirm the first scan results.
2. **Guilt:** As mentioned earlier, guilt is another emotion often found in women who have lost their babies.
3. **Anger:** Even if the abortion happened due to natural causes, the pregnant woman might still develop the emotion of anger. Usually, it is directed toward themselves, their partners, family, Doctors, or even the Supreme power that controls everything. The unfairness they experienced, when compared to other pregnant women, is the cause for anger.
4. **Depression:** Soon after a miscarriage, many women show symptoms of depression that include a disinterest in performing daily activities like eating or sleeping.
They could also display a lack of focus or have trouble making decisions.

5. **Envy:** Another profound emotion that is developed by women who experienced pregnancy loss is envy. This envy is often felt toward expectant parents, and if left unchecked, they might develop a psychotic condition.
6. **Yearning:** A severe and intense longing to be with the baby will develop when the women experience a miscarriage. In some instances, women imagine pampering and playing with babies. Make it a point to discuss your condition with your partner and family members.

Keeping aloof from others will only complicate the situation. The support you receive from your partner and family members is the best space to open up your feelings and emotions. They are the people to whom you can vent your troubling thoughts.

There are several ways through which you could move yourselves to attain proper healing.

1. **Your Decision, Your Right:** Even if you listen to the comments and suggestions of your family members and friends, ultimately, the decision to take up certain activities to enhance the healing process rests upon you. Many people will suggest removing the maternity clothes or baby products you have already collected for the post-maternity period.
2. **Take it Slow:** During the healing phase, make sure to do one thing at a time. Never plan multiple things at the same time and do not plan for the future. The healing phase needs time, and during this phase, you will realize that the mood experienced one day will be different from the other. Your focus should be on how to complete that day's tasks successfully. Also, make sure that you do not make any serious or complicated decisions during this phase.
3. **Give Adequate Care for Yourself:** Try to take enough rest, eat properly, and engage in the different activities happening in the family. The more you engage in the various activities, the faster the healing process will be. Never seek relief in drugs as it will only aggravate the condition. Likewise, if your Doctor has advised you to consume medicines, do so under their guidance.

4. **Keep and Maintain a Journal:** Write down the thoughts and feelings you experience as it might be an excellent outlet to let go of your pain and other emotions.

Another doubt that might pop into your mind would be the appropriate time for planning another pregnancy. Once you have crossed the healing phase and are completely healed from the mental and physical wounds attached to the miscarriage, you can start preparing for the pregnancy. However, it mainly depends on the gestation period when the pregnancy loss happened. If the miscarriage occurred before two months of pregnancy, your body might not have undergone much exhaustion.

Hence, immediately planning for another pregnancy makes sense. However, ideally, it is good to plan the next pregnancy after two-to-three months or after two or three menstrual cycles. It is good to conceive and handle the pregnancy only when your body is fully recovered and you are emotionally fit. You can discuss this with your Obstetrician before planning your subsequent pregnancy and the contraception methods that ought to be followed until then.

Take time to heal emotionally and physically. It is recommended to wait for one menstrual cycle or more before trying to get pregnant again. During future pregnancies, make sure to request frequent prenatal visits for your peace of mind. Even if you are not in a high-risk category, regular visits will enable you to remain calm. Try to be proactive. Try to learn about the different conditions of pregnancy so that you would be able to discuss treatment options with your Doctor. Never compare your pregnancy with another person's pregnancy. No two pregnancies are exactly alike. Above all, stay positive. Even if the discomforts trouble you, always remember that it is part and parcel of your pregnancy. In the next chapter, let us discuss preterm labor and the different factors that lead to this condition.

38

PRETERM LABOR AND DELIVERY

If the baby's birth occurs before the completion of 37 weeks of gestation, it is called a preterm delivery. It can be a spontaneous process or an offshoot of an underlying medical reason that might cause harmful effects for either the mother or the baby. Conditions such as cervical incompetence, growth restriction, insufficient blood supply, placenta previa, placental abruption, unexpected accidents, pre-eclampsia, etc., are some of the possible reasons for a preterm delivery.

However, there are cases where the mother experiences pain and contraction before completing the 37 weeks of gestation, thereby leading to delivery. According to WHO, about 15 million babies are born preterm every year—more than 1 in 10 babies.

Babies born before 37 weeks of gestation are not fully developed, and hence they may need special care in a neonatal care unit. The earlier the birth, the higher the chances of developing health issues in the baby. The preterm baby might have problems relating to breathing and feeding, and they are prone to develop infections as well. Premature birth is one of the primary causes of death of babies under five years of age. Several factors act as triggers for preterm delivery.

1. Previous history of preterm birth
2. Multiple pregnancy
3. Severe infections during pregnancy, like UTI
4. Cervical incompetence
5. Untimely water break
6. Abnormal shape of the uterus

Even though some of these reasons can be identified, sometimes it isn't easy to pinpoint the actual cause for the preterm labor. Another major cause of preterm labor is the short interval between pregnancies. If the interval between two pregnancies is less than 18 months, then the chances of a preterm birth are relatively high for the second one.

Likewise, women diagnosed with uncontrollable gestational Diabetes might also have preterm labor. Pre-pregnancy counseling will help to identify the risk factors for preterm labor. It is often difficult to predict preterm labor by tracking the contractions alone. As you enter the third trimester, you are most likely to experience Braxton-Hicks contractions.

I have encountered many cases where the women do not show any symptoms at all. However, during the routine ultrasound, the shorter length of the cervix might be seen in such cases, suggesting the onset of labor.

I remember meeting Shyamili, who came for her routine eighth-month ultrasound scan. She was perfectly okay and was not expecting delivery any time soon. While performing the scan, I found that her cervical length had reduced to 0.9 cm. I immediately informed her husband, and she was taken to the hospital. Two days later, her husband called me and thanked me for the timely advice.

On her way to the hospital, she started experiencing pain and contractions, and by the time they reached, her water broke, and she delivered two hours after reaching the hospital. As the baby was premature, they kept him in the ICU. If you doubt premature labor, it is good to visit the hospital so that the Doctors will examine you and will do the needful. It can be quite distressing if you are told that you are in preterm labor.

Nevertheless, there are quite a lot of treatment options available to reduce the chance of a preterm delivery. According to your health conditions, your Doctor may prescribe the following:

a) Medicines to stop or slow down the contractions
b) Steroid injections to enhance lung maturation of the baby
c) Antibiotic if your amniotic fluid bag has broken

There are a few treatment options available to reduce the risk of preterm labor. Depending on your risk factors, Doctors might offer the following three options:

1. Wait and watch closely – You will be asked to come for frequent check-ups to measure the length of the cervix to check whether labor is approaching or not.
2. Progesterone supplements – A hormone supplement called progesterone is offered to decrease the risk of preterm labor. It is given as tablets and injections to avoid the risk of preterm labor or a miscarriage.
3. Cervical stitch – This is a surgical procedure where a stitch is placed at the opening of the cervix.

I hope this information is enough for you to understand preterm delivery and what to expect clearly. In the next chapter, let us learn about cervical incompetence, a major cause of preterm labor.

39

CERVICAL INCOMPETENCE

The cervix is the lower part of the uterus, which opens into the vagina. It is otherwise called the mouth of the uterus. The cervix opens at the time of delivery to allow the baby to come out of the uterus.

Cervical incompetence, otherwise known as cervical insufficiency, is the weakening of the muscle fibers resulting in the premature opening of the cervix. You might have already heard about this term, as I have mentioned it many times in my previous chapters. Cervical incompetence, if untreated, might lead to miscarriage or premature labor.

Cervical incompetence mainly manifests at the fourth to the fifth month of pregnancy when the cervix can no longer withstand the baby's weight. I remember meeting Vaishali, a three-month pregnant woman who came to visit me for her ultrasound scan. Everything was normal, except the cervical length. Usually, the cervix should be at least 3 cm in length.

In Vaishali's case, it was 2.5 cm. Her Obstetrician decided to put a suture around the cervix to avoid miscarriage and premature birth. Cervical incompetence is one of the primary causes of recurrent pregnancy loss. Are you aware that such an issue might occur at any time in your pregnancy journey? Cervical incompetence is a clinical and ultrasound diagnosis.

Transvaginal ultrasound is more accurate in diagnosing cervical incompetence. Cervix length less than 3 cm with or without internal os opening is considered cervical incompetence. Sometimes, the internal os would be closed; however, Doctors immediately put a suture if the cervical length is less than 3 cm to save the pregnancy.

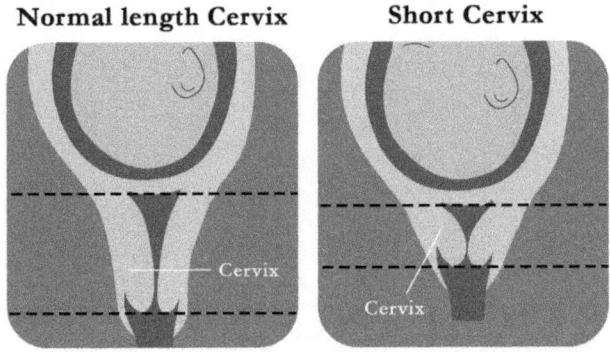

Diagram showing normal and short cervix

Cervical incompetence does not have any signs and symptoms in the early stage of pregnancy; hence, diagnosing the condition is difficult. Watch out for symptoms like pain and heaviness felt in the pelvis, spotting, bleeding, etc.

If detected early, a minor surgical procedure called cervical cerclage is done. The process is a minor day care procedure that includes inserting stitches at the upper or lower portion of the cervix as early as the condition is detected. The stitches support the baby. If cervical incompetence is detected after 30 weeks of pregnancy, then surgery is not advised. Such patients will be asked to be on bed rest for the rest of the pregnancy period. If there is a history of incompetence in a previous pregnancy, cervical cerclage is done at 12 weeks to 14 weeks of pregnancy. Remember, the decision to treat cervical incompetence rests solely with the Obstetrician.

Like cervical incompetence, another major problem you might encounter during the "happy phase" of your life might be an ectopic pregnancy. Let us discuss this condition in the next chapter.

40

ECTOPIC PREGNANCY

Pregnancy is a life-changing phase in a woman's life. It starts with fertilization (the fusion of the egg and the sperm) through sexual intercourse with her partner. This fertilized egg then travels from the fallopian tube to the uterus and gets attached to the endometrial lining. There are some exceptional cases where the fertilized egg implants outside the uterus and grows. This condition is known as an ectopic pregnancy.

In most cases, an ectopic pregnancy occurs in the fallopian tube. I have encountered several instances of tubal pregnancies. Apart from tubal pregnancies, an ectopic pregnancy can also occur in other areas of the body, like the ovary, abdominal cavity, cervix, etc. An ectopic pregnancy causes life-threatening issues for the mother when left untreated. Identifying an ectopic pregnancy is very difficult in some women as they do not present any symptoms.

However, some women show early signs of pregnancy like a missed period, breast tenderness, nausea, etc. Even if you do not have any signs, the pregnancy test will be positive for an ectopic pregnancy.

Warning signs and symptoms become noticeable once the pregnancy starts growing in the wrong place. I recall meeting Sheethal, who complained of light vaginal bleeding and pelvic pain in her second month of pregnancy.

She was overexcited on receiving the news of her pregnancy; however, the vaginal bleeding created confusion, and she immediately went to meet her Obstetrician. Her early pregnancy scan was due, and the Doctor ordered her to undertake the scan immediately.

She approached me for the scan, and I noticed that the pregnancy had occurred in her right-side fallopian tube. I asked her to consult her Doctor as soon as possible. The tension in my voice was palpable, and she recognized a sign of imminent danger. This incident happened at the beginning of my career several years ago, and hence, I was not very confident in dealing with critical patients. That is why I decided to let her Doctor talk about this issue with her.

One of the primary causes of tubal pregnancy is damage to the fallopian tube due to an infection or inflammation. Light vaginal bleeding and pelvic pain are the first warning signs of an ectopic pregnancy. An ectopic pregnancy might result in the rupture of the fallopian tube. In that case, it can be life-threatening for the mother. This condition has to be dealt with immediately by a surgical procedure. The imminent signs of ruptured tubal pregnancy are severe abdominal or pelvic pain accompanied by vaginal bleeding, extreme light-headedness or fainting, and shoulder pain.

An uncomplicated ectopic pregnancy is treated by medication. Ectopic pregnancy is not the end of your reproductive life. Now let us move on to another topic, Rh incompatibility, in the next chapter.

41

RH INCOMPATIBILITY

Rh disease in pregnancy is a common phenomenon that is seen in couples with Rh mismatch. The four major blood groups present in human beings are A, B, AB, and O. All individuals belong to one of these blood groups. Interestingly, each blood group contains a surface antigen based on which the groups are classified as Rhesus positive or Rhesus negative.

This classification is widely termed as Rh classification or Rhesus classification. And hence, we have A+, A-, B+, B-, AB+, AB-, O+, and O- blood groups. If you are unaware of your blood group and the Rh factor, your Doctor will advise you to check it during your antenatal visit.

A significant part of the Indian population is Rhesus positive. Rh factor is crucial in pregnancy as couples belonging to different Rh factors might pose complications to the baby. If an Rh-negative mother and an Rh-positive father conceive an Rh-positive baby, there will likely be issues due to Rh incompatibility or mismatch. The Rh incompatibility might not affect the first pregnancy. However, the problem will arise in subsequent pregnancies. The chances of Rh sensitization are high in cases of miscarriage and ectopic pregnancy, during interventional procedures like chorionic villus sampling (CVS) and amniocentesis, or after a blood transfusion from an Rh-positive individual.

These conditions sensitize the Rh-negative blood of the mother, thereby producing antibodies. These circulating antibodies in the mother's blood will enter the fetus' circulation and destroy the red blood cells of the unborn baby in subsequent pregnancies.

This condition happens especially when the baby's blood group is Rh-positive. However, if the baby's blood is Rh-negative, the antibodies will not harm the baby or the mother in any manner. The complications associated with Rh incompatibility mainly depend on circulating antibodies in the mother's blood.

The milder form of the disease often presents as mild anemia in the baby. However, the severe form of this condition manifests as severe anemia, jaundice, heart failure, and sometimes death of the fetus within the uterus.

Rh incompatibility is diagnosed through a blood test known as Indirect Coomb's Test (ICT). Once the Doctor is aware of your blood grouping and your partner's, and if you are having a second pregnancy, the Doctor will ensure that you undergo this test to avoid further complications. ICT helps understand the levels of Rh antibodies in your blood. Along with the blood test, the Doppler ultrasound scan helps assess the anemia and other complications in the unborn baby.

As newer interventions are available in the medical field, the complications arising due to Rh incompatibility have drastically reduced in the last two decades. As Rh antibodies are the culprits in triggering the issues, treatment is given to neutralize the antibodies. Intramuscular Anti-D injection is given to Rh-negative mothers at the 28th week of pregnancy. If you accidentally miss the injection at this period, do not worry about it. If the Rh status is positive in your baby, the mother will receive an Anti-D injection within 72 hours of the baby's birth. The Anti-D injection helps prevent the production of Rh-antibody in your blood. A baby with Rh incompatibility is also treated depending on the severity of the signs and symptoms. The most common symptom is jaundice, the severe form of which is treated by phototherapy and blood transfusion. Now let us move to another major topic, "the common issues in pregnancy."

42

THE COMMON ISSUES IN PREGNANCY

Once my professor mentioned that discomforts in pregnancy are like the "chutney" you receive with a plate of Biriyani. Even if you do not like to partake of the chutney, it will be served with your main dish.

Similarly, women do not prefer discomforts to accompany their pregnancy. Hence, thinking about getting rid of the discomforts will only intensify the issues that ultimately lead you to more discomforts.

Let us have a look at the common discomforts experienced during pregnancy. Remember, you might not be the only person suffering from these issues. Never feel disheartened if you find yourself devoid of these discomforts. Instead, feel happy for remaining in a pleasant stage.

1. Itching

Pregnant women often experience itchiness. The itching might be over the abdomen or all over the body. I remember meeting a patient who came for her seventh-month scan. I was perplexed to see the tiger stripes on her abdomen.

When asked about it, she replied that she was unaware that rashes often accompany scratching. The itchiness was troublesome, and she did not know how to tackle it. Hot weather, stretching of the skin, dry skin, etc., aggravate itching. Some tips you can adopt to get relief from itching include

    a. Moisturizing the skin with lotions and oils,
    b. Wearing loose cotton clothing,
    c. Avoid scratching, and
    d. Seek help from your Doctor.

In severe cases, your Doctor will advise steroid tablets or steroid ointment for application. Sometimes cholestasis of pregnancy (liver condition) can cause extreme itchiness. In that case, you will be asked to get a blood test (LFT) to know the liver function. The good news is that the itchiness will subside promptly after the delivery of the baby.

2. Leg Cramps

About 50 percent of pregnant women experience leg cramps, which manifest as calf muscle pain or discomfort. It is more common during the second and the third trimesters.

The pain is usually experienced at night and often disturbs sleep. The slow circulation of blood is one of the primary culprits for this condition.

Some tips which help in managing leg cramps:

    a. Drink plenty of water
    b. Gentle massage over calf muscles
    c. Rest your legs on a high raised pillow while sleeping
    d. Take frequent breaks from prolonged sitting or standing postures
    e. Take vitamin D supplements
    f. Seek medical help in case of severe pain. Sometimes clots in the veins (venous thrombosis) cause pain, swelling, and redness in the leg. This is a medical emergency that needs immediate treatment.

3. Varicose Veins

Varicose veins are not uncommon in pregnancy. During pregnancy, the blood vessels bulge as the enlarged uterus compresses the adjacent veins. The varicose veins appear as bluish worm-like or spider-like patterns beneath the skin. It usually does not cause any other symptoms. However, occasionally they cause pain and discomfort in the legs. The varicose veins can be prevented and managed by following the tips mentioned below:

a. Avoid standing for longer periods
b. Rest your leg on an elevated pillow or a stool
c. Exercise regularly
d. Wear compression stockings or socks

Small varicose veins will revert to normalcy after delivery. In such cases, treatment is usually not required for this condition.

43

COMMON INFECTIONS IN PREGNANCY

It is a well-known fact that the immunity level reduces during pregnancy. Hence, pregnant women are vulnerable to infections. Tackling these infections is quite challenging during pregnancy, as pregnant women cannot consume many medicines during this phase. These are some of the common infections encountered during pregnancy.

1. Common cold (Viral cold)
2. Urinary tract infection
3. Flu
4. Typhoid
5. Chickenpox
6. Malaria
7. Rubella and Measles

➤ **Common Cold:** Cold is the most common viral infection that can annoy you during the peaceful phase of pregnancy. The infection is mainly confined to the nose and throat. If you are afflicted with a cough or cold, it might take a week or more to subside.

In the majority of cases, the infection wanes without any antibiotics. The common cold will not have any harmful effects on the baby. However, there are certain cases where antibiotics are offered. If the phlegm turns yellow or green, it is best to take antibiotics after consulting the Doctor. Certain medications are safe to use against the symptoms of the common cold. They are antihistamines, cough syrups, and decongestants. They will reduce nasal stuffiness; paracetamol helps relieve headaches and body aches, and brings down fever. Several home remedies help in tackling the issues associated with the common cold:

- Drink plenty of water to avoid dehydration
- Consume warm beverages
- Steam inhalation soothes the nose
- Add a pinch of salt to hot water and gargle frequently

➢ **The "flu" (Influenza)**: The influenza infection caused by the H1N1 virus is also known as Swine flu. Compared to the symptoms of the common cold, the symptoms of Swine flu are slightly more concerning. The signs and symptoms of influenza include fever, body pain, tiredness, headache, and sore throat. Since the virus causes the flu, the treatment is similar to that of the common cold. Usually, paracetamol tablets are used to relieve the symptoms.

➢ **COVID-19 Infection:** We are passing through the greatest pandemic of the century, the COVID-19 pandemic. Several studies showed that pregnant women are equally susceptible as non-pregnant individuals to acquire Covid-19 infection. Pregnant women are advised to take utmost precaution from getting afflicted by Covid-19. Here are some of the practical tips you could follow to prevent yourself from contracting this disease:

1. Follow social distancing while moving out in public places.
2. Use face cover to protect yourself.
3. Drink plenty of water to stay hydrated.
4. Eat a healthy diet, as it might help boost your immunity, enabling you to fight against many issues and infections.
5. Take vitamin supplements to boost immunity.

6. Make sure not to miss your Doctor's appointments and regular antenatal scans. I have witnessed many women who missed their Doctor's appointments and relevant tests, citing that it was unsafe to visit a health care facility during the pandemic.

Current evidence suggests that there will be no harmful effect on the baby if the mother is afflicted with the COVID infection. As per WHO guidelines, all pregnant women are encouraged to get COVID vaccination, which is safe at any stage of pregnancy. The vaccine is also safe if you are breastfeeding.

> **Diarrhea (Watery Stools):** Diarrhea is one of the common issues during pregnancy. Usually, it is treated without the help of antibiotics. If the condition is accompanied by fever and blood or mucus discharge in the stools, it can be assumed that it is a bacterial infection.
> In case of bacterial diarrhea, antibiotics and probiotics are prescribed. Some of the remedies for diarrhea are listed below:

- Drink lots of fluid
- Avoid spicy food
- Antacids, antidiarrheals, antiemetics, and antispasmodics will help to reduce the symptoms

> **Chickenpox Infection:** Chickenpox manifests in the form of fluid-filled blisters on the skin surface. The blisters usually start appearing over the abdomen and soon spread all over the body. It is a highly contagious disease that spreads from one person to another. Antiviral drugs that should be taken for seven days are often administered to patients suffering from chickenpox.
> Chickenpox afflicted patients are isolated from others to prevent cross-infection The chance of spreading the infection will be high till the crust is formed, and once it is formed, you are no longer a carrier of the disease.
> Varicella-Zoster immune globulin vaccine can be taken to protect against chickenpox infection. The good news is that chickenpox infection usually does not affect your baby.

> **Urinary Tract Infection (UTI):** Did you know that UTI is the most common infection during pregnancy? The physical and hormonal changes in pregnancy make the urinary tract vulnerable to infection. Some of the common symptoms of UTI are a frequent urge to pee, inability to completely empty the bladder, and burning sensation and pain while passing urine. Sometimes, it is difficult to differentiate pregnancy discomforts from UTI. If left unchecked, UTI might pose complications to the mother and the baby. You should be aware of the several tips that help you to prevent UTI.

   a. Consume a good amount of water and fluids.
   b. Empty your bladder during every washroom break.
   c. Clean the pelvic area after peeing.
   d. Use disinfectant on the surface of the closets before and after peeing.
   e. Consult a Doctor to get treatment in the early stage of the infection.

44

FIBROIDS

Fibroids are non-cancerous muscle lumps in the uterus. They are very common in women during the childbearing age. They are classified as mural, subserosal, and submucosal based on their location in the uterus.

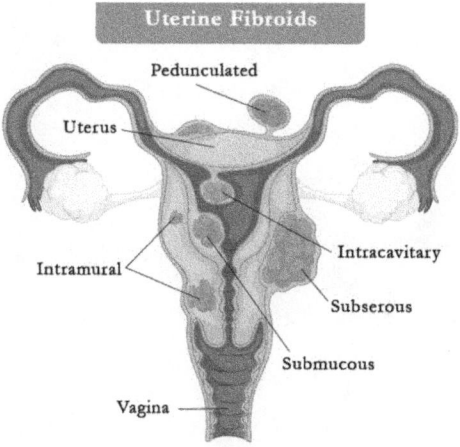

Fibroids are harmless, and they will not disturb the pregnancy in a majority of cases. The signs and symptoms of fibroids depend on their location, size, and number in the uterus.

In 60%–70% of cases of pregnancy, the fibroids are asymptomatic and do not change in size. However, pain is the most common symptom of fibroids, especially with large fibroids.

The fibroids which are seen within the uterine cavity are called submucosal fibroids. The large submucosal fibroids can cause miscarriage and infertility issues. Other rare complications of fibroids include preterm labor, bleeding, malpresentation of the baby, and excessive bleeding after delivery. The acute pain associated with the presence of fibroids is due to red degeneration. I recall meeting Shivani, a pregnant woman who came to my clinic. She was nine weeks pregnant and was experiencing severe pain in the pelvic area.

As the pain started to increase, she suspected a miscarriage and rushed to the Doctor. The Doctor could not diagnose the cause for her pain. After the ultrasound scan, I revealed that Shivani had a large fibroid in the uterus that had undergone degeneration. The first question I encountered was about the survival of her baby. I comforted her and said that her pregnancy was safe. I still remember her smile breaking out amidst the tears upon hearing my words. It is vital to realize that fibroids grow in one-third of all pregnancies due to the effect of the estrogen hormone.

I hope you are now acquainted with the condition of having fibroids during pregnancy. Now, let us examine the issue you might encounter if you become pregnant after 35 years of age.

45

GETTING PREGNANT AFTER 35 YEARS

Getting pregnant after the age of 35 is not a rare incidence. Whatever may be the reason for late pregnancy, there are certain pros and cons associated with it.

Let us see how pregnancy and pregnancy outcomes differ in younger ages and after 35 years of age.

- Age and fertility are indirectly proportional. Aged women find it difficult to conceive due to declining hormones and aging eggs.
- The risk of congenital disabilities in offspring born to elderly women is higher—the risk of Down syndrome increases as the age of the mother increases.
- The risk of miscarriage is higher due to chromosomal abnormalities in the embryo.
- The chances of multiple pregnancies are higher. This condition can be attributed to the infertility treatment they undergo, like ovulation induction and IVF.
- The chances of developing PIH and Gestational Diabetes are higher in an elderly pregnant woman than in a younger mother.

- The prevalence of placenta previa (abnormal placental location) is higher.
- The chances of having a stillborn baby are doubled.
- Incidence of preterm labor and delivery is relatively higher by 20 percent.
- An elderly mother has a greater chance of giving birth to a lower-weight baby.
- Difficult labor and chances of C-section are higher due to weak contractions of the uterine muscles.

Despite all these issues, prenatal screening tests like blood tests, ultrasound scans, and amniocentesis help to ensure that the pregnancy outcome is fruitful, even in the case of elderly mothers. The table provided below contains the details of the potential risk of carrying babies with genetic abnormalities as age progresses.

Age of Mother	Risk of Baby with Down Syndrome	Risk of Baby with Genetic Problems
20	1 in 1667	1 in 526
25	1 in 1250	1 in 476
30	1 in 952	1 in 385
35	1 in 250	1 in 192
37	1 in 224	1 in 127
39	1 in 136	1 in 83
40	1 in 100	1 in 66
42	1 in 63	1 in 42
45	1 in 30	1 in 20

CONCLUSION

You have now reached the final chapter of the book, where I would like to provide you with some inputs on Happy Parenting. If you are a first-time parent, do not be afraid, as every parent has passed through your stage before becoming an expert in the area of parenting.

Sometimes, it is not easy to define or write about parenting. However, I will attempt to write about happy parenting and how you can enjoy the phase of parenthood from the experience that I have had being the father of two daughters.

Taking care of a baby is one of the most challenging and interesting jobs with many responsibilities. Do not be afraid as it is also a highly rewarding job. However, I have seen many parents approaching this phase without the constant focus that they ought to have on the whole.

Our parenting techniques are often born out of our gut feeling or we imitate the parenting methods of our parents. We never check whether these techniques are effective for raising our babies. It is astonishing to realize that parenting is one of the most researched and studied subjects in the field of humanities. If you ever encounter any doubts or issues while raising your baby, it is always good to seek advice from the elders and your Doctors.

I happened to read a book titled *The Ten Basic Principles of Good Parenting* by Laurence Steinberg, the famous American psychologist. He has excelled in the field of adolescent psychology and has provided many theories on how parents should raise their children in a better manner.

The 10 principles that he has provided on good parenting are based on findings from 75 years of research on parenting conducted in the field of Social Science.

He comments that good parenting helps foster emotions and qualities such as cheerfulness, kindness, honesty, self-control, empathy, self-reliance, courage, and cooperation. Above all, good parenting also helps in promoting intellectual or rational curiosity in children; it motivates them to learn new things and creates an unending desire to gain success. Good parenting has also protected children from developing antisocial behavior, anxiety, alcohol and drug abuse, eating disorders, and depression.

Let us take a close look at the parenting tips that Laurence Steinberg provides.

1. **What Matters is What You Do**:

Children imbibe behaviors from their parents. Behavior is mostly an imitative process more than a genetic function. That is why Steinberg says, "What you (parents) do makes a difference. Do not react on the spur of the moment." Instead, ask yourself what you want your child to become and try practicing that behavior yourself. When children find their parents following a certain behavior, they will imitate it. According to Laurence Steinberg, this is one of the primary principles that needs to be followed.

2. **You Can Never Be Too Affectionate**:

Steinberg comments that while excessively loving a child is not harmful, providing too many material possessions in the place of love can be. Hence, make sure that you are affectionate to your children, but at the same time do not give them too many unnecessary things.

3. **Always Be Involved in Your Child's Life**:

Getting involved in your child's life is time-consuming and needs hard work. It also involves rearranging and rethinking the priorities that you have in life. Once you become a parent, your priority might be your baby, and sacrifice becomes one of the primary mottos that you need to uphold in your life.

Always make sure to be with your children mentally and physically and listen to their needs whenever they call for you. However, note that "being involved" does not mean taking up the child's homework. Homework is a technique that the teachers often use to re-check whether their students have understood the concepts taught. If parents become too affectionate and write the homework for their children, the teachers will never know if the student has learned the concept.

4. **Change Your Parenting Style According to Your Child's Behavior:**

Your parenting style should be in tune with your baby's development. That means the parenting techniques should vary according to the age and development of the child.

5. **Make Sure to Set Rules:**

Setting rules really matter. If you cannot manage your child's behavior, especially when they are very young, you might experience a hard time in the future managing them. That is why the elders always comment, "pick them early." However, setting rules should not be misread as micromanagement. Once they start growing, every parent should make it a point to let their children make their own choices.

6. **Enhance Their Independence:**

An offshoot of setting rules is to enhance the child's independence. With set rules, they will learn to develop proper control and self-direction. In fact, independence and self-direction are the two major tools every child needs to succeed in life.

7. **Be Consistent:**

If you set rules, make sure to stick to them rather than varying them day by day. Rules should be enforced every day and not enforced intermittently. Hence, if your child misbehaves, it is solely your problem and not your child's. Consistency should be your primary disciplinary tool.

8. **Stay Away from Severe Disciplinary Methods**:

Parents should avoid harsh disciplinary practices such as hitting and using abusive language. These harsh techniques would only lead to added misbehavior on the children's part. Steinberg adds that "there are many other ways to discipline a child—including 'timeout'—which work better and do not involve aggression."

9. **Make Sure to Explain Your Rules and Decisions**:

Parents should explain the rules and decisions they have made regarding their children. This will create a sense of belongingness in the children, and they will understand that they are needed. They will also understand the expectations that their parents have placed on them.

10. **Be Sure to Respect Your Child**:

You should treat your child with respect. They will learn the quality of respect when the same quality is offered to them. Make a note to listen to their opinions, and ensure that you speak to them politely.

I believe that these tips will help you in raising a better child. I wish my readers all the very best in their parenting process.

I would appreciate any feedback from the readers. Your suggestions will help me finetune my upcoming editions.

You can send your suggestions and feedback to sunilkumar@addonhealthcare.com.

Happy Parenting!

MY NOTES

REFERENCES

The content in this book is verified from below mentioned resources:

1. Ultrasound for obstetrics : https://fetalmedicine.org/
2. Ultrasound for obstetrics and gynecology:https://www.isuog.org/about-us.html
3. Good Clinical Practice Recommendations on Preconception Care:https://www.fogsi.org
4. Routine Antenatal Care for a Healthy Pregnancy:https://www.fogsi.org
5. Corona(COVID- 19) infection and Pregnancy : https://www.rcog.org.uk/coronavirus-pregnancy
6. Best Clinical practice considerations for Obstetrics and Gynecology:https://www.rcog.org.uk/guidelines
7. Patient information leaflet: https://www.rcog.org.uk/en/patients/patient-leaflets/
8. Your Pregnancy and Childbirth: A guide to pregnancy from the Nation's Ob-Gyns:https://www.acog.org/womens-health/your-pregnancy-and-childbirth
9. Pregnancy Centre:https://www.webmd.com/baby/default.htm
10. What to expect when you are expecting:https://www.whattoexpect.com
11. Newborn care:https://www.whattoexpect.com/first-year/newborn/

Some of the popular Pregnancy Apps for your mobile phone

1. Pregnancy and baby tracker WTE
2. Baby Centre - Baby tracker
3. Pregnancy and Due date tracker
4. Ovia Pregnancy

ABOUT THE AUTHOR

Dr Sunil Kumar G.S., is a renowned Bengaluru based Radiologist with more than fourteen years of professional experience. Dr. Sunil obtained his MBBS degree from Yenepoya Medical College, Mangalore in the year 2006; his MD degree in Radiodiagnosis from Siddhartha Medical College, Tumkur in the year 2010; DNB degree in Radiodiagnosis from the National Board of Examinations, New Delhi in the year 2011; and FRCR from the Royal College of Radiologists, London in the year 2013. Dr. Sunil has previously served as the Consultant Radiologist at Fortis hospital, Bengaluru.

With his expertise in Fetal Medicine and Woman and Child imaging, he founded the "add-on Scans and Labs" in 2016, which became a centre of excellence for 'Women and Child Health.' He has offered his services as a guest faculty at various medical and non-medical conferences. Dr. Sunil also has the credit of being the author of the book *Set the Ball Rolling*.

www.ingramcontent.com/pod-product-compliance
Lightning Source LLC
Chambersburg PA
CBHW032356040426
42451CB00006B/31